A BODY MADE TO WIN

Optimizing
the Body's Natural Defenses
to Heal Even from the Deadly COVID-19 Virus

JOANN LOVE, M.D.

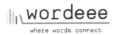

where words connect

A BODY MADE TO WIN

Optimizing
the Body's Natural Defenses
to Heal Even from the Deadly COVID-19 Virus

A BODY MADE TO WIN: Optimizing the Body's Natural Defenses to Heal Even from the Deadly COVID-19 Virus

First Edition
ISBN (paperback) 978-1-946274-70-0
ISBN (eBook) 978-1-946274-71-7

Library of Congress Control Number: 2021941544

Jacket design: Okamoto
Interior Design: Amit Dey

Published by Wordeee in the United States, Beacon, New York
Website: www.wordeee.com
Twitter.com/wordeeeupdates
Facebook: facebook.com/wordeee/
e-mail: contact@wordeee.com

ADVANCE PRAISE FOR
A BODY TO WIN

Dr. Love offers several concise resources to maintain optimal health for this trying time as well as going forward. It is clearly written based on her many successful experiences as a medical practitioner. She describes through contextual rigor how to go beyond the confines of traditional medical avenues with proven suggestions to strengthen our self-healing immune system.

—Dr. Kenneth Silvestri, E.D., CCH
Systemic Psychotherapist
Author, *A Wider Lens: How to See Your Life Differently*

Dr. Love has been a thyroid guru for many years now...patients not only love her but prefer her when it comes to any thyroid issue. This is her passion, and patients benefit from it.

—Ricardo Rubio, M.D

"Dr. Love draws on her decades of clinical experience as a complementary health pioneer in developing her insightful and proven protocols. Designed to strengthen and balance the body's innate immune and energy systems, her no-nonsense approach goes beyond theory to offer practical solutions for working *with* the body to help individuals take charge of their health.»

—Jim English
Science and Health Editor, Author

DEDICATION

For all who taught me and continue to teach
me how to live well.
And to those who serve during the pandemic
with selflessness and courage.

TABLE OF CONTENTS

FOREWORD

by
Dr. Paulette Moulton, M.D.

I had the pleasure of meeting Dr. Love over 35 years ago. Given we are both physicians, we immediately had a shared understanding of the importance of health and healing. It wasn't until we got to know each other better that we realized that our similarities in our approach to wellness are even more profound.

Western medicine is the framework in which we both trained, but at some point in our practicing medicine, both of us realized that the true fundamentals of medicine are much more "unconventional" than we had been taught. Eventually, our medical careers became significantly less Western as we incorporated more holistic, integrative elements of healing in our practices. While integrative medicine is becoming more mainstream, physicians who stand behind holistic practices remain few and far between.

Dr. Love is an experienced and established physician who has worked in medicine for many decades. She has been exposed to medical practice in multiple locations, not only in the United States but around the world. It is not without significant experience that she shares with us her knowledge and expertise.

In this book, she illustrates for her readers how the human body is made to win. This book is especially timely, given the

COVID pandemic. The relevance in this moment is striking as we enter our second year battling the novel Coronavirus.

The world's smartest physicians and scientists have yet to find a treatment option that is reliable for combating this viral illness. This is why relying on our own bodies is of utmost importance at present. In her extremely important piece of work, Dr. Love gives a compelling recipe for how we can each optimize our body's natural defenses in order to heal from ailments. By the end of this book, you will be equipped with an armamentarium of tools to ensure that you use your innate powers and allow your body to be "A Body Made to Win."

INTRODUCTION

This book has been written by a doctor, albeit an unconventional one. I believe conventional medicine is one of man's greatest advancements, but it does not supersede everything. In conjunction with the body's natural ability to self-heal, conventional medicine could be most powerful in optimizing health for a body already made to win. Unfortunately, Western medicine has been overpowered by Big Pharma at the cost of undermining the body's natural defenses to heal us.

The past year-plus has shown that medicine does not have all the answers despite its many advances. A pandemic, COVID-19, has caused our medical system to buckle and initially baffled our scientists. Worldwide, it has impacted all of us in one way or another, whether we got the disease or not— loss of loved ones, loss of work, isolation, mental fatigue, loss of health even after recovery and the list goes on. As we learn more about this 'Beast' of a virus, I'm sure various medicines will be developed to prevent or manage it more effectively. As of this book's writing, several vaccines have come to market to combat the deadly novel pathogen, but there'll always be another. So, the best way to protect ourselves from harm is to maintain optimum health that allows the body to win the fight against disease.

Many super strains of bacteria we're faced with today have been created by the very medicine we've used to treat them.

When an organism becomes resistant to a drug, it mutates because it, too, has survival instincts. As long as we exist, new pathogens will come along to challenge us. Let us hope none like COVID-19 for another few centuries or beyond.

This book is a guide for people who believe the human body has the power to heal itself. The information and recommendations found herein focus on the body's ability to recover and survive from anything threatening its well-being. Since COVID-19 has been a major disruptor to the world and to me, I have used my battle with the 'Beast' to illustrate how a body built around a robust immune system can avoid or minimize the effects of any threat, infection, or other insults on its own without unnecessary medical intervention.

A healthy body is all-powerful, and many healthy people have withstood the virus. Let's put in perspective the reality of COVID-19 casualties: 97% to 99.5% of people infected with the virus recovered on their own.[1] Of the people hospitalized, many had other medical conditions: 93% of the people who died of COVID-19 in the USA had underlying conditions, such as asthma, heart conditions, obesity, and vitamin D deficiency, etc.[2] Still, it should also be noted that healthy people became severely ill with the disease and had to be hospitalized; some died, and others have developed Post-Acute COVID-19 Syndrome or Long Haulers as it is called among the lay public. An estimated 10% of patients are dealing with prolonged illnesses resulting from the virus: brain fog, headaches, shortness of breath, fatigue, and loss of or distorted sense of taste and smell, among other debilitating challenges.[3]

My wish for every person who suffers from post-COVID-19 syndrome is that a knowledgeable caregiver can help him or her navigate the advice given here and that they'll find helpful information in this book on how to heal their bodies and aid their recovery.

For people looking for natural alternatives to healing, this is where a doctor like me comes in. Again, I'll use my COVID-19 recovery journey as an example to explain how body systems work in healing and recovering from illnesses. Most of all, this book is truly about how to optimize health, which always begins with a great immune system, best supported by a healthy diet and exposure to sunlight. A healthy body will win.

About Me

I'm Joann Love, M.D., owner-operator and staff physician at the Hot Springs Wellness Clinic located in Truth or Consequences, New Mexico.

After suffering from a nasty bout of COVID-19, I introduced a new three-week program to aid patients recovering from this clever, opportunistic virus based on what I did to recover. If you follow the advice found here, one that works with your body's natural immune system, you'll likely fast-track your recovery and regain your health.

Currently a spa doctor, I spent a decade working in emergency medicine, followed by two decades working in preventive, occupational and urgent care medicine. Twice during my career, I have been a private practitioner, first as a general practitioner and decades later in an Anti-Aging practice. A born naturalist, always searching for alternative approaches to conventional medicine, I've worked on Native American reservations, including Rosebud and Pine Ridge in South Dakota. In the winter months, chasing the sun so vital to my health, I've worked as a cruise ship doctor to the Caribbean and Hawaii. I've also studied medical hydrology at the International Society of Medical Hydrology and Climatology in Europe with renowned spa doctors as disease is not what interests me, but the recovery from disease—a spa doctor's specialty.

At the beginning of the AIDS epidemic, I was a resident in medicine at Lincoln Hospital in the South Bronx, New York. Having been exposed to the then 'disease of the century,' I understood infectious diseases better. For a year and a half, I also studied tropical diseases in St. Croix while working in the emergency department. As an emergency room doctor, I've seen patients from the point of view of different medical specialties: trauma, pediatrics, dermatology, urology, etc., and I've treated people in all stages of life, from delivering babies in the emergency room to attending to end-of-life patients in their last hours. I've seen conventional and nontraditional medicine practiced from all angles and in many countries throughout my career. I know I have something to say.

As happens with most naturalist physicians, it is expected there might be some pushback from the conventional medical community. Still, I'll share my thirty-eight years of knowledge and experience of what has worked for many of my patients and me. You will decide your medical journey, which I hope will be based on common sense. Undoubtedly as you read this book, you'll find out just how incredible the human body is and how you can heal your own body.

As a general rule, I don't recommend or place people on lifelong medications (except for missing hormones) unless there is absolutely no other choice, which is rare. My focus is on helping patients recover their health to the point where medications as a lifestyle option can be discontinued. My role as a physician is and always will be in the pursuit of optimum health for others and myself.

My Journey into Medicine

I knew something was wrong. I chronically suffered from recurrent low-grade fever, chronic fatigue, undiagnosed hypothyroidism, celiac disease, which meant feeling sick if I ate flour, and a recurrent urinary tract infection in my early twenties. None of the twenty-two doctors I consulted could figure out the root cause of my illness. As is done in so many cases, they treated my symptoms by prescribing antibiotics for my abdominal pain and urinary tract infections, which caused me to develop a leaky gut and a worsening of my low thyroid function. I was miserable. No, I was a wreck and couldn't accept or imagine living my entire life feeling that lousy. What would be the point?

My illness continued to worsen. Listlessly, I laid on my couch for six months, which I found entirely frightening. Then slowly and miraculously, I'd started to feel better. This was the way I wanted to feel every day. As I had before, I knew I would relapse if I didn't figure out what was causing this intermittent flare-up of blahs.

As it turned out, much of what I'd experienced stemmed from the result of an incomplete yet painless root canal that had become chronically infected. How many months and years could I have had optimum health if any of the twenty-two doctors I consulted had figured it out? Had they even tried to probe to find out what other than my symptoms could be going on within my body, I would have felt better.

Something seemingly so benign as an infected tooth flare-up had overpowered my body.

There had to be a better way to help people, and I wanted to find it. So, it was in search of my health that led me to become a doctor. Then, as now, conventional medicine didn't have all the answers and doesn't seem ready to find them. I studied medicine in Spanish at the Universidad Central del Este in the Dominican Republic. I had to push myself to the brink to learn the complicated discipline of medicine in a foreign language. But the experience was exhilarating, fascinating, and ultimately liberating. It also gave me a clinical advantage and a new language. I speak Spanish.

During my thirty-eight years of clinical practice, I've seen several alternative approaches to helping the body recover its health, from natural herbs, "old-time" remedies to traditional Chinese medicine (TCM), acupuncture and natural therapy. Each has worked wonders in healing people without Western medicine.

One day my tooth broke. A dentist in Chicago, where I was doing an externship, informed me that I had an abscess in my root canal, and I immediately knew this had been the root of my problems. A second root canal was performed, and just like that, I was made whole again. Imagine something so insidious as an infected tooth was as debilitating as any chronic illness. I believe with my whole heart that toxicity from an infected root canal can ruin your life. After all, the body is interconnected.

Because I believe in an educated patient, I want to refer you to the astonishing documentary *Root Cause*, the movie on YouTube. Its release on Netflix created quite a stir in the dental community, enough to have it removed. Not only does it make sense, but it also stands on sound reasoning; the body systems are interconnected. That systemic consequences from an infection anywhere in the body will affect other systems is absolute. So why would an infected root canal be any different? I began to wonder, could this kind of infection account for some chronic illnesses that seem to have no cause? It's a question I ask my patients, and so should all doctors who deal with patients with chronic diseases.

It's the Norm

Most of the time, if one is chronically ill, doctors may never know the true underlying cause of the disease. Could it be that conventional medicine is only too happy to treat symptoms rather than cure diseases? It's a sad reality but often right. The nature of Big Pharma as fix-it-all product makers is a frightening proposition. The truth is that many naturally occurring medicines are hijacked by Big Pharma, synthetically altered, and dispensed to meet "demand." Too often, it's all about money. Instead of taking Valium, one might wander out to their garden, pick some St. John's Wort, and make a calming cup of tea with zero side effects. In comparison, six months of taking Valium have been associated with the early onset of Alzheimer's. According to a Harvard study, taking it (Valium) longer than six months can increase your risk for dementia by as much as 84%.[4]

In my work over the years, and with exposure to patient's treatment in conventional and nonconventional medicines, I found several ways to help patients and myself maintain optimum health without falling prey to the medical-industrial complex. I first assess and correct any hormonal deficiencies, particularly with the thyroid, a master gland that controls all body functions. Out of sync, it causes hyper or hypothyroidism, leading to a whole host of other problems.

Second, I assess whether patients have the nutritional capacity to help the body when in need? If no, I change the patient's nutritional status through diet and supplements. If yes, this means they have been doing all the right things to help keep their immune system stay in tip-top shape. Thirdly, I focus on the number three essential of our therapy: Vitamin D, a vital part of the equation. In my practice, the fourth thing I do is prescribe cannabis to help people wean off synthetic medications for insomnia, anxiety, depression, and pain (certainly, we've heard about the opioid crisis with OxyContin). Instead of helping people maintain their illnesses, my goal is to help them recover their full health naturally by calling on the body's defenses to heal itself.

A side benefit of the changes patients tells me they experience, especially with cannabis, is that it helps manage their insomnia. Insomnia is a major insult to the body maintaining homeostasis. It is the number one reason why I use cannabis indica (CBD/THC) too. I never advise my patients to do anything I wouldn't do to my own body in my practice of medicine. But each patient must decide on their health choices.

The Elephant in the Room

There is an argument that we are all different and, as such, require different treatment solutions. Let's end that now, right here. We are not. If not every one of us, the grand majority, irrespective of race, color or creed, get the same illnesses. We can argue that our environment plays a significant role in our health, and I will not minimize the power of the environment, nutrition, or conditioned belief systems to impact health. Still, metabolically and physiologically, our bodies are built exactly the same way, and we all have the same ability to fight diseases.

We will discuss this more later in the book. But did you know that the third most prevalent illness in the USA is hypothyroidism? Much like the number one and two diseases, hypertension and elevated cholesterol, thyroid disease is common to all races. Because insufficient thyroid levels influence both hypertension and elevated cholesterol, we could even argue that thyroid dysfunction could be the number one disease in the USA. It is so common that I, and most of my family, many of my friends and patients also have it. An astonishing 12% of the U.S. population will have a thyroid disorder, and 60% of that population will have thyroid disease and not know it.[5] So, why would a medical system that pushes pills not treat thyroid conditions, possibly the country's true number one disease? I'll let you decide. In my practice, I always recommend that my patients order a home spot testing kit to assess their thyroid health as they appear more accurate than the commonly done routine thyroid testing, which frequently comes back as normal. A normal test usually means the patient will be denied thyroid hormone replacement.

The thyroid, the little butterfly gland at the base of the throat, is a MASTER gland. It controls and influences a lot of what happens in the body. Consider thyroid hormone the overseer of energy. Lots of thyroid hormone in the system means being in a super energy state. A lack of thyroid hormone means utter exhaustion. The most common complaints caused by inadequate thyroid hormones read like a laundry list: fatigue, hair loss, brain fog, weight gain, hypertension, obesity, feeling chronically cold, elevated cholesterol (leading to heart disease and heart attacks), atrial fibrillation (leading to congestive heart disease), pneumonia, heavy menstrual bleeding, infertility in men and women and Alzheimer's. In children, ADHD, ADD, autism, frequent colds and infections, obesity, depression and anxiety, bipolar disorder, acne, and more are all under the gland's influence. The thyroid's function is vital to metabolism, yet to adequately treat thyroid disease, as I've heard a doctor say, "Would financially break the 'system'." Ask yourself if this is a system you want to have to depend on alone for your health. Should anything else matter but your health?

The Questions We Ask at Our Spa, Hot Springs Wellness Clinic.

Until 1950 this town was called Hot Springs, the City of Health, because of its natural healing waters and almost year-round sunlight essential for vitamin D exposure. Our Spa programs are holistic and are for patients looking for alternative methods to healing from chronic or acute illnesses. At the Hot Springs Wellness Clinic, we address the body holistically as an intricate, intelligent, integrated system. After patients are faced with an illness, we ask, how do we put the body back into homeostasis/balance and, even more important, how to prevent a breakdown in the future? Of course, we prefer that the body is never out of balance.

Maintaining a body in homeostasis, especially in our society today is not an easy task. So, we recommend regular "maintenance check-ups" to keep the body running smoothly. We invite our patients to come back once a year for "tune-up" and detox. We don't think twice about maintaining our cars; why not our bodies, which, by the way, is simply an intelligent machine.

In providing a supportive, healing environment for patients, our primary focus is boosting the immune system. Once a patient arrives at our facility, I will thoroughly analyze their thyroid hormone status. Apparently, thyroid function has been disrupted by a COVID-19 infection, and I agree with the new CDC guidelines for "Long COVID Patients" that include a work-up of thyroid function. However, I request different lab tests, as it is my experience that the CDC recommends TSH and free T4 testing, which will come back as normal most of the time, when in fact, the patient is hypothyroid. I find that blood spot testing done from home is more accurate, so we send patients a blood spot home test kit and evaluate their status according to the results.

Our holistic approach includes a review of health complaints, diet, weight, and the supplements taken. I will also assess complaints related to low hormone levels, sleep habits, exercise routine, time spent outside, activity level and adjust accordingly. Next, we introduce heliotherapy (safe sunlight therapy) and heat therapy from natural hot springs bathing, loaded with minerals and trace elements the body requires. The precise point of this book is to fix the energy system, which is provided by the hormone thyroid. For a more detailed understanding of our six points of service, visit our website.

In general, choosing wellness of all body systems is hard work, and I will tell you it won't be easy. We'll teach you how to make wise health choices in everyday life, which will lead to greater overall health. Making as many changes as needed to get healthy, especially if the body is out of control, has to be done. Understanding how the body works may spark an "aha" moment, and in my opinion, you must understand your body to help it fight the good fight against diseases.

That is what we do at Hot Springs Wellness Clinic. We teach, and we heal. There is no "cross your fingers" and hope attitude in my practice. We believe and have the utmost faith that a body, treated with respect, will wake up and run right. It will win! As a general rule, we believe in the educated patient— one who prefers to work in harmony with their body and in tandem with their provider. We also believe that informed patients will make wise choices for their well-being

CHAPTER ONE

THE VIRUS, THE 'BEAST'

COVID-19 is scary. According to history, it has caused the tenth pandemic since 430 B.C, when typhoid took out a third of the world's population. The last pandemic was recorded a century ago with the outbreak of the Spanish Flu, which killed over 50 million people and infected a third of the world's population, making the COVID-19 pandemic tame in comparison.

COVID-19 arrived in 2019, and everything about this virus is complex, including its dubious beginning. Seven coronavirus strains have infected humans in the past and have been responsible for the common cold and the outbreaks of SARS and MERS. Most of these viruses are not dangerous. Though COVID-19 belongs to the well-known coronavirus family of viruses long familiar to immunologists and infectious disease specialists, it behaves differently. This mutant form of the virus SARS-CoV-2, aka COVID-19, a new strain identified in December 2019, is deadly.

Initially, B.1.1.7, the Alpha variant, was the culprit of the early infections we saw ravaging the world. The virus has since mutated multiple times.[6] As of this writing, seven strains have emerged with even greater efficiency to infect. Some of the new strains are associated with an even more virulent form of the disease. The older strains that seemed not to have infected the younger population have given way to a new strain which does. The newest, more virulent Delta strain currently on a rampage worldwide has arrived in the United States and is attacking the vaccinated and unvaccinated, including younger people. However, it appears that the vaccines are holding up against the Delta variant in vaccinated people and in cases of breakthrough infections, people seem protected from the severity of the disease and death.

Nearly a year and a half into the pandemic, the world is still unsure of the pathogen's origin or where it will end up and how many lives will eventually be lost. At the writing of this book (July 2021), COVID-19 has claimed over 4,196,672 million lives and counting worldwide, a fifth of them in the US.[7]

How the Virus Works

COVID-19, much like the rest of its family, attacks the respiratory system and can cause lower and upper respiratory tract infections spread by person-to-person contact. The stealth virus latches its spiky sugary protein to the ACE2 receptors of the upper airway and the lungs. Once it invades, it hijacks the cells and takes command. If infection occurs, symptoms may appear 2-14 days later, but a carrier may never show any signs or symptoms of the disease. Infection can trigger what is described as a cytokine storm. This means that the immune system, trying to destroy the virus, releases inflammatory proteins into the bloodstream. If the antibodies overdo it, an autoimmune-like behavior occurs where the body literally attacks itself. This can potentially cause inflammatory proteins traveling in the bloodstream to kill healthy cells and organs.

A shutdown of many body systems, leading to death, can occur if this happens. One of the phenomena we've seen with people who've been severely infected, slightly infected or showed no symptoms at all, is post COVID-19 Syndrome or Long Haulers, as it has become known. This itself may primarily be an autoimmune disease that is triggered by a virus.

At the onset of the pandemic, there was mass confusion around the disease's signs and symptoms, and our knowledge was sketchy. As a result, much valuable time was lost in its diagnosis, and because we lacked testing power, the pernicious virus spread rapidly. A year plus later, the symptoms have been identified as:

- Fever
- A dry cough
- Shortness of breath sensation; Trouble breathing
- Fatigue
- Fever with chills and sometimes shaking
- Body aches/rash
- Headache
- Sore throat
- Congestion/runny nose
- Loss of smell and taste
- Nausea
- Diarrhea.

Recently India has been struck by the new Delta variant now detected in over ninety-eight countries. This strain seems more prevalent in the younger population and presents with classic symptoms of a runny nose and fever that seems like a bad cold. According to The World Health Organization (WHO), the Delta variant quickly became the dominant stain worldwide and is the "fastest and fittest" because it is more infectious. I suppose other strains will be arriving to challenge us further.

Consider yourself in an emergency if you:

- Have trouble breathing
- Have persistent pain or pressure in the chest
- Confusion or brain fog
- Blue tinged lips or face
- Inability to stay awake

COVID-19 Smacked Me Around!

Why COVID-19 smacked other victims and me around was due to its cleverness. Outwitting us all, it possesses several mechanisms to elude its host's immune system while learning how to circumvent the body's normal protection. First, it's stealth and undetectable for 2-14 days. By then, it is an entrenched infection way before the immune system knows it's there. Unlike the flu, where the body produces mucus and a productive cough, in two-thirds of the COVID-19 infected cases almost immediately, this virus presents with a dry cough, a runny nose being an infrequent feature. A third of the time, it may produce a cough with mucus production, which might fool us into thinking it's a common cold.

The mucus, coughing and productive phlegm that usually accompany a common cold or the flu, along with a fever, is the body's usual way of dealing with and getting rid of a virus—their purpose is to stop the virus from further invasion and it is also a transport vehicle for antibodies. When the human body finally becomes alert, it's under attack from the COVID-19, it tries to corral and outsmart it, but the clever coronavirus has already begun to do its damage. It has now presented itself as a full-blown, deadly infection. That is why medical workers have called it the "Beast." It is continually infecting others in those 2–14-days with its stealth approach.

I was Sick, and I Knew It.

When all the commotion about the virus started, I told myself that everyone would get this, but I won't. However, I was clearly under an illusion because I forgot to include the word "novel" in my thinking. Novel COVID-19, which means brand new, had never been seen before.

I was working in a cannabis clinic, helping people obtain cards to legally use cannabis as a medication, something I support 100%. So, in a small office, I sat across the desk from patients, some of whom were seriously ill. They may have cancer, chronic pain, degenerative and autoimmune diseases, and COVID-19! At 69 years old, as I have always taken care of my health in every way, I thought I was healthier than almost every 70-year-old I'd encountered.

When I came down with it, I was embarrassed. It meant my immune system didn't give a damn. No matter how many past common coronavirus colds, rhinoviruses or cases of the flu I'd been exposed to in my 69-years, it didn't recognize this nasty bug for a week until it was deeply entrenched in my lungs. My alarm bells went off. I have COVID-19.

I attributed my infection to one of my patients in poor health, only to later learn there were carriers among us. Wait! Maybe my exposure could have been to a healthy person (a carrier) or even the child who came in with their mother. A carrier is someone who has the disease but may never show any signs or symptoms of it yet are highly contagious. Just by breathing out the virus, they are walking lethal weapons. This is one reason why protective gear is such an important part of the disease's prevention. The following week they shut the country down, and I was still coughing.

In late February 2020, my journey with the virus started with a sore throat, not too bad for a day, followed by an occasionally spasmodic cough, which I misdiagnosed as seasonal allergies. Almost nine days later, on March 2, I sat straight up in bed at 3 a.m. in a coughing fit. "What in the world is this?" I wondered.

The 'Beast' is a heck of a coughing infection. It was coughed to 219 countries and territories in a flash. The virus virtually went worldwide by means of coughing, sneezing, breathing, and talking on planes, boats, cars, subways, etc. With only a dry cough, I coughed myself into exhaustion with this puff-puff cough for days and weeks and only once did I cough up phlegm. With no protective layer of mucus or productive cough present, it invaded furiously. Even the constant weird shortness of breath feeling I experienced had its purpose. It's another of the virus's clever survival mechanisms. It forces us to continually take deep breaths and exhale the virus, exposing others by the simple act of breathing or talking.

Unlike many viral infections, COVID-19 infection is usually accompanied by a low-grade fever instead of the high fever one might expect with the flu. This is because fever is yet another of the body's defense mechanisms that the virus circumvents. Having removed some of the body's natural mechanisms to fight it off, the virus invades the respiratory and gastrointestinal tracts. It also has the audacity to invade the heart, kidneys, pancreas, gallbladder, brain and blood vessels, creating blood clots and rashes. Last and most importantly, it attacks the thyroid gland, our master energy system.

> *The 'Beast' knocked me down. I was sitting in a chair or lying down for five days with a fever almost two and a half degrees over my normal body temperature, which would not have qualified me for emergency care as it didn't hit the CDC's 100.4 mark. Because of my hypothyroidism, my body temperature is naturally low.*
>
> *The non-stop, incessant coughing, unless I was using cannabis indica, an old cough remedy, had me prostrated. In retrospect, having read the horror stories from other COVID-19 victims, including health care workers younger than I, I noticed there were many things I knew not to do and things I did that I believe helped. Unfortunately, I'd missed the first signs of the disease because I didn't feel sick.*

> *Much of my emergency room and urgent care work had been centered on treating people who had colds or the flu. I used my years of experience in treating flu and colds to treat my infection. The first rule has always been, GET OUT OF THE IMMUNE SYSTEM'S WAY in that context. Do not interfere at all. Get it optimized and boost it.*

I've spent thirty-eight years advising patients that the fastest route out of a viral infection is self-care. My advice centers on the idea that our bodies have the healing cycle down: attack→repair→restore, but it must be allowed to do the work. Our job is to figure out how best to support our defense system and, most importantly, how not to block and interrupt the attack→repair→restore cycle.

Vaccine or No Vaccine

Like many doctors and providers in the same line of work, I could treat hundreds of influenza cases in a season without contracting it. I hadn't had a cold or flu in twelve years, which is bragging rights, because I was a part-time urgent care doc for much of that time. The only flu vaccine I ever got was during the 1976 President Ford initiative to inoculate the entire country against the swine flu, Influenza A virus, which ultimately led to one death and hospitalized thirteen people. My friends dragged me to a basketball auditorium in a frenzy of fear where the inoculations were being given. Resisting to the very end, I finally overcame my desire to flee the scene and took the vaccine.

The linkage between autism and vaccination in children may stem from maternal hypothyroidism and maternal vitamin D deficiency. According to research, a hypothyroid mother is four times more likely to cause autism in their offspring. It is possible then that the reason some infants fare poorly with vaccines is because these babies, hypothyroid like their mothers, have systems too inefficient to clear the different components of the vaccines, which negatively impacts them. [8]

Because I'm beyond fearful of having that infection again, in fact, positively shudder at the thought, I felt it prudent to take the COVID-19 vaccine. I took both injections of Moderna. Like in the 1950s, there's a push to vaccinate us all. The U.S. is hopeful that most Americans will be vaccinated soon and that herd immunity will be achieved. According to the CDC, "The vaccine has some effect when layered with natural immunity." [9] Let me stress the layered with natural immunity here.

With each virus mutation, which can change the sequences of proteins, one only hopes the vaccine will be effective against future strains. Recently, a few fully vaccinated people have been getting what is known as 'breakthrough infections,' but fortunately, they are not experiencing the severity of the disease. The most recent deaths from COVID-19 are from people who have not been vaccinated. Your primary care physician is a good person with whom to discuss your options. If you are a high-risk patient, definitely follow your doctor's advice.

Sneaky, stealthy, clever, changeable, deadly, this virus is not to be taken lightly. It has brought the world to a halt. Science is fighting the good fight, and with a winning vaccine, we can hopefully put this pandemic behind us. The great news is that the vaccine is proving beneficial to some Post COVID-19 syndrome patients (Long Haulers) who, after taking it, have either recovered their health or showed improvement in many of their residual symptoms.

CHAPTER TWO

BODY BUILT TO HEAL
AND SURVIVE—WHAT COULD
REALLY BE GOING ON?

There is a little-known syndrome, Euthyroid sick syndrome (ESS), associated with higher levels of the little-known hormone, Reverse T3 (rT3). Known as the hibernation hormone, rT3 has been recorded at elevated levels in hibernating animals, and so it seems with us too. A high rT3 level is believed to activate a protective state for a body in severe distress by shutting down its energy resources to help it survive. This happens in famine, trauma, severe infections, burns, anorexia nervosa and other dire assaults on a body that needs to conserve energy. When this happens, rT3 (Mayocliniclabs.com) acts as an energy-blocking thyroid hormone that blocks active T3 thyroid hormones' ability to produce cellular energy.[10] I mention this because I think this may very well be the condition related to the pervasive malaise experienced by Long Haulers of the COVID-19 disease. In hindsight, when I felt chronically ill, I believe rT3 syndrome might have been in play as my body focused all its energy on controlling the infection in my abscessed root canal tooth.

Commonly misdiagnosed, rT3 is often called Chronic Fatigue. In addition to the CDC's recommendation re: thyroid workup for Long Haulers, I recommend all cases of Long COVID Syndrome get their rT3 levels measured, particularly those who are bedridden, as these patients may have developed Reverse T3 syndrome. The Long Haulers may also have developed a second form of thyroid disease, a form of hypothyroidism, Hashimoto, where the immune system attacks the thyroid gland, often requiring thyroid replacement. Check for Hashimoto's hypothyroidism by getting a full thyroid panel workup, including a blood test for anti-thyroid antibodies, TPO and rT3. If these tests come back as normal, take note if the numbers for Free T3 and Free T4 hover at the bottom of the range, "almost low."

It has been noted that the thyroid gland is negatively affected by a COVID-19 infection. In 15–30 percent of hospitalized cases, the patient's lab work is consistent with Euthyroid Sick Syndrome—low Thyroid Stimulating Hormone (TSH) and T3 and an elevated rT3. Is it possible then that a COVID–19 infection has been so traumatic that the body puts itself in survival or hibernation mode and blocks T3 energy by producing rT3 to conserve energy? Reverse T3 syndrome would undoubtedly explain this change. Could it also be that after a severe attack of the virus, unfortunately, the body does not or cannot revert to a more active thyroid hormone state once the crisis has passed, so feelings of fatigue and brain fog persist? Medical literature regarding rT3 syndrome is sparse, so it is difficult to conclude its full effect on the body. However, this should underscore the need to pay attention to impaired thyroid function following a COVID-19 infection. There are lab tests for rT3. Request the full panel of thyroid lab tests: TSH, rT3, Free T3, Free T4, TPO antibodies if you have concerns about your ongoing malaise.

A Plausible Theory on Fatigue in Long Haulers?

Does an educated guess beat the "We don't know what is causing this" answers we usually get from the medical establishment about chronic fatigue experienced by Long Haulers? The CDC indicates a thyroid workup should be done on these patients. The question we must ask is, what are we seeing from the test results? Is it Hashimoto, the common disease, or rT3 syndrome? Is reverse T3 syndrome real?

My sense says we are seeing two disease processes here, both caused by a malfunctioning thyroid gland after a COVID infection. The common Hashimoto is an inflammation of the thyroid gland that affects the production of thyroid hormone. It causes fatigue, weight gain, puffy face and slow heartbeat. Patients with persistent symptoms of hypothyroidism can drag themselves to work, but those who have rT3 Syndrome, who are so severely ill, can barely manage to leave the couch because of the extreme state of malaise, along with other hypothyroid symptoms. Can sunlight bathing help wake up the hibernating state as it does other living things every spring? Will the other modalities listed here to strengthen the thyroid hormone system also create energy? How do we persuade the thyroid gland to produce T3 for energy and stop its conversion to rT3?

It is accepted in the medical literature that reverse T3 is sometimes elevated in chronic fatigue syndrome. Are those with chronic fatigue syndrome who also have autonomic dysfunction, Postural Orthostatic Tachycardia Syndrome (POTS, racing of the heart and feeling faint from just standing up) also in the hibernation state? Is it intentional that the body forces us into sleep to aid in its recovery? If this is true, there is little focus in the medical community on persuading the body to revert to normal T3.

To check for the rT3 syndrome, see a provider and request a lab test for Reverse T3, along with the full panel, TSH, Free T3, Free T4, and TPO antibodies. Accurate blood tests hopefully will enlighten us on how to help these patients. However, remember, I would check a home test kit first, as all five tests are available in a blood spot thyroid panel. If rT3 is low, follow these recommendations on strengthening your thyroid naturally and see if you can be treated with a T3 replacement such as Cytomel?

So, when faced with this runaway viral infection—an infection that would unleash millions of antibodies over the next few days, weeks or months, I went to work bolstering my immune system with vitamins, minerals, healthy foods, and the most important, the hormone, vitamin D. I knew that in the case of COVID-19, the body produces millions (if not billions or trillions) of new B cell antibodies specific to the coronavirus. Besides, there is a spike in helper T-cells. How can I assist them and not inhibit their production and process was my main concern?

What will I eat or avoid eating to boost the immune system? What should I take for the puff-puff, constant dry cough? What will help the burning chest sensation produced by the cytokines-storm our immune system liberates during an attack? These are essential questions to ask. (See chapter, "Steroids to the Rescue, But Beware.")

I also engaged with the idea of what role sunlight and vitamin D should play in my battle and recovery? An adequate supply of thyroid hormone is needed to produce the energy to power through the attack. How can I boost and not block thyroid production?

I recommend that you, too, should familiarize yourself with the body's self-preservation abilities. When I compare my case to the experiences of people who became seriously ill, I told myself something, "You sure were lucky for being unlucky." Years of taking care of my immune system, even though I was unlucky to get the damn thing, meant my body was able to work under the best conditions, which made me lucky and a survivor.

CHAPTER THREE

A BODY BUILT TO HEAL: MAKING IT WORSE—REDUCING THE FEVER IS A FOOL'S FOLLY

Most of the time, COVID-19 infection is accompanied by a low-grade fever, so keep it that way. Initially, according to the World Health Organization (WHO), taking Ibuprofen with a COVID-19 infection was a bad idea.[11] It was believed to worsen the infection by elevating the ACE receptors, which the Coronavirus uses to invade! Later they reversed themselves on the subject, but I'll stick with the original advice because it supports common sense.

I hope you're not the patient who reaches for medication bottles the moment you realize you're getting sick. Just because you can lower a fever and do something to make yourself feel better doesn't mean you should. I get it that the muscle aches and pains that accompany a COVID-19 infection are annoying, and yes, Ibuprofen will help with that, but do you really want to help the virus invade further for a little more comfort?

Contrary to popular belief, fever is a part of the body's defense mechanism to protect itself. A fever helps to eradicate the virus and is an essential healing signal for antibody production. It influences the immune system, both innate and adaptive, including the neutrophils' and macrophages' ability to regulate T and B antibodies to fight off the disease.

If you are popping antipyretics such as aspirin, acetaminophen, naproxen, and Ibuprofen to stop the fever, all the way, you'll be fighting the body's mechanism to protect and heal. While you're loading up on meds to stop the fever, the virus is freely and happily invading the body. The implication is that you've now potentially turned a minor infection into a worsening infection.

As long as the fever does not reach dangerous levels that denature the body's protein (105.8 degrees Fahrenheit), try to give it as much opportunity as possible to play its vital role.[12] If your fever increases to dangerous levels between 103-104 degrees, immediately contact your health provider for options and, if necessary, temporarily use medications to bring down the fever. Physicians at the Royal Society of Medicine in London do not recommend that patients lower their fever at the beginning of a COVID-19 infection, and neither do I.[13] A secondary reason noted in the article is that when a fever was lowered in certain upper respiratory infections, viral shedding, including the coronavirus-19, increased. It is just what the world does not need, more coronavirus floating in the air.

Here is another point to keep in mind. If you take medications to reduce fever at the onset, the immune system could fight back with a rebound fever, going even higher than it would have in the first place. Why? Because you've permitted more virus activity and the body must now work harder, and now you'll be taking medications every 4 hours to lower the higher fever you have induced. The 'Beast' is smart, and possibly during the intervals when you've lowered your fever, there is also less antibody production. Remember this: The Mayo Clinic thinks a fever is harmless and probably helpful and advises not to treat it until it is above 103 degrees Fahrenheit.[14] Fevers in children should be watched carefully, and if over 101, my advice is to treat it.

I read a medical doctor's account of his severe COVID-19 infection. I was utterly perplexed when he wrote that his wife bought him over-the-counter drugs (OTC). I wanted to know which ones! I'm glad he recovered. I read another account of a woman who'd been sick for fifty-two days and took Tylenol and Benadryl every six hours for the entire time. I wanted to say, "Stop that!"

My approach is: If the body wants fever, it gets a fever. To treat my fever, I did what a patient I encountered some twenty years before did. I drove the fever higher. This patient entered the infirmary on a cruise ship I was working on somewhere around the middle of the Gulf of Mexico, with a fever of 104. With no lab or x-ray available and only a urine analysis kit, I prayed that her fever was from a urinary tract infection. As it turned out, it was. When I repeated the temperature reading a few minutes later, it had dropped to 101. I inquired if she'd used Tylenol to lower the fever before coming to see me as it seemed to be "kicking in." She said: "No, I was so cold and shivering I got under all the covers I could."

That day I learned the meaning of fever chills. It's the immune system seeking help to drive the fever up by making you feel cold. Naturally, if you're cold, you'll find a way to feel warmer even in the presence of a fever. The fever and chills persuade you to bundle up. If you have a very high temperature accompanied by extreme shivering, treat them and consult your doctor. Otherwise, tough it out because fever is your friend.

The CDC's temperature of 100.4 as the cutoff to detect a potential COVID-19 infection is beyond ridiculous. For me, that would only be over 3 degrees of fever.[15] My normal body temperature, due to hypothyroidism, is 97.2, and with the COVID-19 infection, I saw it go as high as 99.8. Normal body temperature is 98.6, so I had what would have appeared to be a very low, low-grade fever. According to the CDC guidelines, I could have been in the throes of a full blast infection but still would not have been detected as having a fever and an active COVID-19 infection. I'm not alone.

Hypothyroidism, as mentioned, is one of the most common diseases in the USA, so many low-temperature people are walking around who could have an active COVID-19 infection but would not be detected as having a fever when in reality they do.

If you feel cold while having a fever, my advice is, crank up the heat literally by getting under blankets periodically, and if it doesn't push your body temperature over 103, go for it. If you see the fever approaching the danger zone of 104 degrees Fahrenheit or, as recommended by The Mayo Clinic, 103, temporarily lower it in a cool bath, take your favorite antipyretic and contact your provider. You may have pneumonia. Remember, all hands-on deck, this COVID-19 is a bloody awful battle to fight. So, be brave when possible and leave the big baby "I just want to feel better stuff" behind.

If you find the symptoms unbearable, I recommend using cannabis indica for chest discomfort and cough, and it will also help you sleep. Choosing a high CBD/low THC strain with an extra boost of CBD is a phenomenal sleep aid, and it will likely reduce lung inflammation as it does in laboratory rats.

I felt some chills early on in my battle with the virus. So, I did what the fifty-year-old cruise ship patient did. I got under the covers and shivered. Lucky for me, I'm in the desert, so I could also be in the sun. As for the baths, I live in a house attached to a hot spring Spa and took frequent baths. The water temperature was 107.6, so I didn't stay in very long, finding it too physically stressful. The fact is I used heat therapy effectively during my infection.

My illness confined itself to my lungs, and there is no evidence of lung damage. I can still swim but haven't returned to running because it seems like too much. Maybe I'm refusing to recognize how brutally I was affected, but I will know the truth when I begin to run again, if ever. I think my brain function survived intact, too, you might agree, or I couldn't have written this book.

CHAPTER FOUR

FURTHER ENLIGHTENMENT ON
HOW TO MAKE IT WORSE

A constant dry cough was the first thing I noticed about my infection. It seemed that the cleverest way COVID-19 differs from and is superior to the cold-causing coronavirus and that of other respiratory infections is in its ability to suppress the immune system's response. Its superior contagion ability is because it persuades the body's response system to skip the river of protective mucus usually produced during a case of the cold or the flu.

The COVID-19 cough is as dry as the Chihuahua desert where I live in New Mexico. In a 28-day illness, from start to finish, I coughed up phlegm on just one occasion. Patients with COVID-19 who show flu-like symptoms may use drying allergy cold and flu medications. Like treating a fever, this is a bad idea. These medications will dry you out. Not quite the approach recommended by Harvard Medicine, or me, or anyone whose healing method is based on common sense and has a full appreciation of the miracle called the human body.

With a typical cold or flu, the cough rounds up the mucus, viruses, and bacteria and expels them by coughing and expectorating. The congestion is caused by inflamed blood vessels, and though terribly annoying, this blocks more of the nose surface to prevent further viral invasion. Each of the symptoms, the cough, the congestion, the runny nose, headache, fever, tiredness, aches, and pain, etc., are part of the body's immune response to kill the virus. People may think the virus causes the miserable condition they are experiencing, and indirectly that is true, but the reactions are from the immune system trying to kill the virus that causes the symptoms.

By blocking the immune system with cough suppressants, decongestants, antihistamines, and fever reducers, we inadvertently inhibit the immune response and allow the virus to super invade. It may sound counter-intuitive that a medication sold to make you better is making you worse, but my experience has shown that to be the case. Again, I am inclined to ask, isn't it just pharmaceuticals treating the symptoms?

Most of my patients who couldn't shake a viral infection like the flu or who develop a secondary bacterial infection from opportunistic organisms were taking these over-the-counter quick-fix remedies. This is always why I ask my first question, remember? "What did you do to make it worse?"

It's not hard to turn a cold or flu or COVID-19 infection into a secondary bacterial infection, sinus infection, bronchitis, or pneumonia that will require a visit to the clinic, x-rays, antibiotics, and missed work. A three-day cold has become a three-week cold because the immune system was prevented from doing its job. Z-Pak will work with the secondary bacterial infection but does nothing for the virus. The problem: antibiotics knock out gut bacteria, paving the way for leaky gut and weight gain noticed a few months later. The question that begs an answer is: while battling the virus, does interfering with the gut's ability to uptake nutrients and further depressing the immune system a good idea?

Do you remember the sage advice given by top doctors on how to treat the flu? "Chicken Soup." Which means OTC medications won't work. I give the same advice; however, make the chicken soup with rice. Noodles made with flour are out as gluten can provoke an antibody attack on your thyroid gland. In the early stages of the flu, Tamiflu, a prescription-only drug, an antiviral that attacks the virus, can prevent it from multiplying and offer relief. Depending on your age and state of health, if you get the flu, I suggest you spare the office visit where you might be exposed to COVID-19 and request a telemedicine visit instead. Additionally, follow the natural healing advice found here as it applies to all viral colds and flu illnesses. Some good news: influenza, the usual viral infection we suffer yearly, has dramatically declined due to mitigation patterns and the use of masks.

At the onset of the pandemic, without fully understanding the illness at hand, what were doctors doing? They were prescribing antibiotics for a bacterial infection that didn't exist and wouldn't work on a coronavirus. COVID-19 and most other upper respiratory tract infections are usually viral in origin. However, secondary bacterial infections may occur, and as I said, Z-Pak may be prescribed. Let me repeat: antibiotics do not treat viral diseases.

Unfortunately, antibiotics increase the risk of developing one of its common side effects, Clostridium Difficile, a diarrheal illness that follows powerful antibiotic treatments. In Italy, this severe diarrheal illness contributed to the death of many elderly patients hospitalized with COVID-19. Imagine working on a patient on a ventilator with severe diarrhea or worse yet be the patient? The question to ask your physician about prescribing any powerful antibiotic treatment must be: do I really and honestly need this Z-Pak or Steroids? Ask it. Ask it of yourself and your doctor.

I've had patients who come into my office with a viral infection and fully expect a prescription of antibiotics. Based on my personal experiences, patients will work over their doctors until they get one prescribed. So, please don't hold it against providers who prescribe them, for they fear patients' sizable wrath. I want to repeat and stress, Z-Paks work on bacteria, not viruses!

I also advise my patients to ask a second question: "What can I do to help myself?"

My answer: "Why not get out of the way, and let your body kill this virus?"

No doubt, the pandemic has overwhelmed the already overburdened medical system. Every time a patient runs into the doctor's office for a minor illness, the body can resolve; they are burdening the medical system. Doctors already work under time constraints and don't have enough time to thoroughly diagnose illnesses because their offices are filled with people who can help themselves by using their common sense. Having to defend their services to insurance companies further robs doctors of time. You have to become a smart patient.

I maintain that my advice is correct regarding the "Beast." This brings me back to the COVID-19 cough and the merciful effects of medicinal cannabis indica and CBD (see the chapter on cough). When I first read about patients who were Long-Haulers, I went to the website Body Politic. It was there that I noticed three things; the main disease they had was asthma. Only a small percentage of them used cannabis—more used alcohol. The main medications used were inhalers and Tylenol. This does not surprise me, especially alcohol consumption, acetaminophen use, or the fact that they had asthma.

I wondered if vitamin D, selenium, zinc, iodine and vitamin B12 deficiency, vegetarianism, alcohol use, any history of a root canal and undiagnosed hypothyroidism were among other prominent contributing factors to the body's long haul to recovery? I'm always advising against vegetarianism, especially with a lethal infection, and you will see why in the chapter, How to Feed Your Immune System.

CHAPTER FIVE

MAKING IT BETTER—THE COUGH, LESS LUNG DAMAGE, CANNABIS AND CBD

I am a physician with a personal dislike of chemical-based medications. I encourage patients to take natural herbal medicines whenever possible.

> *During my illness, I turned to what I consider the most remarkable herbal medication, cannabis Indica. I took a 10 mg dose of cannabis indica in a tincture twice a day to treat my persistent cough. I am here to tell you it worked very well. Though I still had the burning sensation behind my sternum—breastbone, the sensation of shortness of breath, malaise, low-grade fever, the coughing dropped to a minimum. After taking THC/CBD, I would still feel like I wanted to cough, but the cannabis effect relaxed my chest, and the cough just didn't happen. That is when I said, "Wow, smart, miraculous herb."*

In 1785, the genus of cannabis was described by Jean-Baptiste Lamarck. He identified two strains, cannabis sativa found in east Asia and cannabis indica found in the Kush Mountain region of Afghanistan. The biochemistry of each THC and CBD has different effects. CBD (cannabidiol), a non-intoxicating compound, has medicinal healing power and can alleviate anxiety, pain, and inflammation. It becomes more potent in the presence of THC (tertrahydrocannaboid also a cannabinoid). However, the full spectrum cannabis plant with a boost of CBD from the hemp plant may provide the most relief for the cough and lung inflammation.

Until the 1930s, cough preparations contained cannabis indica syrup. Current cough preparations on the market are made with synthetic chemicals and even narcotics to achieve a similar effect to cannabis. In my view, they are imposters. Cannabis sativa, which also has medicinal benefits and cannabis indica, had yet another benefit in COVID-19; both have resin with antiviral properties. The jury is out whether cannabis depresses the immune system. There is evidence both pro and con. However, given that a COVID-19 infection can cause massive inflammation and CBD is helpful in this aspect, it is worth seeing if there are beneficial effects.

THC and CBD have traditionally been used for cough, and so far, the research is encouraging.

To me, cannabis is a wonder drug. Still, it is a drug, and I'd use less rather than more. In hindsight, I wish I had been using a CBD boost along with the THC/CBD because of its anti-inflammatory effects. Taking CBD has been proven to help people recover from the lung damage caused by the coronavirus-induced cytokine storm. Taking THC/CBD with a CBD boost is recommended, and I also recommended it for the Long COVID Patient during their recovery.

Cannabis, used medicinally for 4,000 years, is one of 50 herbs that are the basis of ancient Traditional Chinese Herbal Medicine. A study from Israel indicates that CBD and the terpenes found in cannabis are two times more effective than Dexamethasone in dialing down the dreaded cytokine storm of COVID-19 in the lungs.[16] CBD studies have also shown that it helps increase interferon productions, a protein that activates the production of immune cells. Cannabis can also prevent viruses from replicating, all while decreasing some of the annoying symptoms of the infection, namely cough, pain and the anxiety that runs high for most people infected with COVID-19. So, what's your pleasure, Dexamethasone, a prescribed steroid or cannabis?

A recommendation, if tolerated, is to take THC/CBD 10 mgs every 6 to 8 hours with a boost of 10 mgs to 100 mgs of CBD during the most acute phase of the infection and recovery. In general, use a sativa cannabis during the day, a hybrid in the evening and an indica for sleeping. If you have never used cannabis, you may want to take one-half of the dose or 5 mgs or lower every four hours to see how it affects you. Remember, CBD works more efficiently if THC is present. You will be boosting the medicinal part of the plant, increasing its therapeutic effect.

I've been a cannabis consultant for the past seven years, and I can tell you it is the best medicine I have practiced. Certainly, in view of the fact that American medicine is credited with being the third leading cause of death in the USA, that's a big deal. The toxic effect of some medications prescribed today is causing new problems for already ailing patients. Just read the list of side effects, and they should have you running for the hills and who can forget OxyContin.

Our goal at Hot Springs Health and Wellness is to treat the root cause of diseases, but we also want to manage and relieve patients' signs and symptoms as naturally as possible. The use of cannabis, if indicated, is a part of the treatment approach at Hot Springs Wellness Clinic.

> *I thank cannabis indica for drugging me into sleep, alleviating my cough, and making my chest burning sensation more bearable. As for the shortness of breath sensation, nothing I did helped. I ordered a bronchial inhaler from the pharmacist, but it didn't improve my shortness of breath, so I dropped it. I lived with its annoying presence in my life. Finally, after weeks it went away. Even now, seven months since the onset of my COVID-19, I cough easily, and I cough more, but not like the first few weeks following my illness when everything, as the virus intended, made me cough.*

CHAPTER SIX

MAKING IT BETTER—
THE PULSE OXIMETER
FOR OXYGEN LEVEL

Blood oxygen levels indicate how well the body distributes oxygen (O^2) from the lungs to the cells. Typically, it's done through what is known as an ABG TEST. Most O^2 levels are at a saturation between 95% and 99%, usually between 75 and 100 millimeters of mercury. Potential COVID-19 patients admitted through the hospital E.R.'s triage department and have pulse oximeter oxygen levels of 95% to 100% are usually sent home. However, as Loyola University Medical Center noted, there are cases where patients present without respiratory distress but have low oxygen saturation and are in great danger. This has become known as happy hypoxia seen in COVID-19 patients.[17]

When the lungs are compromised in a COVID-19 attack, it's a good idea to monitor oxygen levels as hypoxia (low blood oxygen) can, as stated above, become a problem. If quarantined at home, an excellent way to monitor oxygen levels is through a pulse oximeter device. It should be noted here that the pulse-ox is quite reliable when oxygen levels are high but less so when oxygen levels are low. Regardless, invest in one by buying it ($20 and as low as $9) from an online store if you are on lockdown. If someone in the family already has one, use it to monitor your oxygen levels. If you aren't clear on what the pulse oximeter is, it's a gizmo in doctor's offices that is slipped onto your finger and gives a reading of your pulse and blood oxygen levels. To properly use the device, place the pulse oximeter against the finger pad of your index or middle finger (no fingernail polish, please) and wait for the reading to calibrate. One number is your oxygen level, the other your pulse.

> *Nothing was more reassuring to me during those critical days of my illness than looking at the pulse ox on my finger and seeing that my oxygen level was stable. I would feel increasing shortness of breath, and I was sure that my oxygen level was falling, only to be pleasantly surprised that my (O^2) oxygen level was unchanged. I would relax immediately, just to feel a few hours later that I was getting worse and discovering again that my oxygen level was unchanged.*

Checking O^2 levels hourly is a reasonable guideline given the nature of the virus. Those who have underlying conditions that compromise breathing functions, such as anemia, congestive heart congestion, asthma, COPD, etc., should watch their oxygen levels even more closely. It's a good idea for patients who suffer from any of these conditions to know their baseline oxygen number anyway.

Always exercise caution if oxygen levels are falling. If the oxygen level drops below normal on the pulse-ox, pack your bag. It's an indication you'll need to be seen in the E.R. Hopefully, there, you'll be treated with high-flow oxygen therapy and not a respirator. Please don't feel too anxious about that respirator because doctors are using them less frequently now. If blood oxygen levels stay stable during the infection, at your baseline, try to ride out this disease safely at home. Soon, as opposed to what is available now, an effective antiviral will be available for COVID-19, similar to Tamiflu for the flu.

Here is another good reason not to run to the doctor or provider should you come down with COVID-19. You might be the patient who infects them! More than 3,600 medical workers have died in the USA since the onset of the virus. Now thanks to the vaccine, our health care workers are protected. You would do well to skip the emergency room or clinic unless there's an absolute need to be there. Those who tend to panic at getting a cold and feel compelled to bring it into the urgent care facilities or family practitioner office, please don't. We've talked about that. Here is the reality. In the United States, 1.8% of people infected with COVID-19 will die of the disease, and another 10% of those will show signs and symptoms of the Long-Hauler syndrome. Chances are you will recover naturally.[18]

If you believe you have been infected, do venture out to a testing center where, from the car, you can be tested with little exposure to others. The good news is in the fall, with just one test, a COVID-19 swab will also include testing for the flu.[19] If your influenza test is positive, see a provider to get on Tamiflu if indicated. If your COVID-19 test is positive but not life-threatening, follow my advice. If your flu and COVID-19 tests are negative, but you have a persistent upper respiratory infection, and you're older than 65, ask your provider if it's prudent to test for the Human Meta Pneumonia Virus.[20] This test is similar to that of COVID-19 in that it is a nasal swab, and PCR testing is considered the gold standard of virus detection. The results may take a few days, but a doctor's visit may be necessary.

On the third night of those five challenging first days, I felt increasing shortness of breath and noticed my oxygen level was falling slightly, from 95 to 93 percent. It was late in the evening. I'm a doctor and need to know when to use all medical options available. If my holistic treatment was failing, I needed to be in a place with emergency care should I need it.

"Might be going to the ER for a little oxygen," I told myself. "When it drops to 88%, I'll have to go. I might be going on a respirator, steroids, and antibiotics, and I might not ever be the same. I might even have to call an ambulance, and this may be how I could die." I remember telling myself to get up and pack some things. If I would be hospitalized, I needed to get it together. Burdened under severe malaise, I heard myself say, "No way. I can't get out of this bed. Oh boy," I thought, "here we go."

I focused on the B-antibodies, specific to this infection in my chest and told them, "Whoa, don't overdo this, you'll kill me, and if I go down, you'll go down too." I knew the danger could be real because of two things; what I was feeling was my immune system battling the virus. I have an autoimmune disease, Hashimoto's, causing hypothyroidism. Not good. Then something resonated and profoundly said, "You're almost 70. You have an autoimmune disease; you could die of this. Let the immune system do what it has to do." And that point, I mentally got out of the way of my immune system.

What I have repeatedly noticed since then is that so many people have said the same thing. "I was so sick I thought I was going to die." Some must have thought like me; I'm too sick to be able to get up and go to the hospital. As a consequence, they passed away at home. In NYC early in the pandemic, the home deaths went from an average of 35 daily to 200 daily, and of course, there were other casualties caused from people with chest pain who were too afraid to go to the Emergency room for fear of contracting COVID.[21]

Regarding the pulse, which is the other number the pulse oximeter reads, remember this: with each degree of fever, the pulse goes up by 8.5 beats.[21] With a temperature of 99.8, 2.6 degrees, over my usual body temp of 97.2, I was up 21 beats a minute to a pulse of 98. No problem, I told myself. A normal pulse is around 72 beats per minute. I decided to wait it out and watch the oxygen level, not the pulse. Of course, if I had a racing heart over110 beats, I would have immediately acted on it, as it could be a sign of pneumonia.

CHAPTER SEVEN

STEROIDS TO THE RESCUE —BUT BEWARE

As I mentioned earlier, in non-life-threatening cases, natural remedies can help manage the disease. For example, according to the Medical College of Georgia researchers, CBD will help decrease lung damage and inflammation.[22] Conventional medicine's treatment approach for lung damage management and inflammation is steroid therapy. But here's the catch. Steroids knock back antibodies and open the body up to secondary infections. From the Chest Journal literature, we know the incidence of pulmonary fungal infection has increased in recent years and appears to be related to the use of steroids in chronically ill patients. [23]

In COVID-19 patients, many suffer pulmonary inflammation. If you can stand the burning sensation, the shortness of breath and the dry, constant cough that comes with the virus, as with a fever, live with it. But be careful and vigilant because the immune system can kill you going after the virus with a cytokine storm. If steroids are indicated on an emergency basis, don't resist. Steroids are known to decrease the storm and death rate in hospitalized patients. If this is where you end up, don't be in denial about it and follow your provider's advice. Nothing good comes from being a COVID-19 denier, particularly if the lungs are compromised.

Steroids are hormones naturally produced by the body. There are three types: Anabolic-androgenic such as testosterone, minerocorticoseroids produced by the adrenal glands to influence salt and water balance, and glucocorticosteroids such as cortisol are anti-inflammatory. In a healthy body, they are regulators. Synthetic corticosteroids such as Prednisone and Dexamethasone are given when the body's immune system overreacts, and they do help patients with severe symptoms of an overactive immune system. Cases such as skin diseases, arthritis, and asthma are examples. Doctors who prescribe steroids in acute immune flare-ups will wean the patient off them slowly to prevent adrenal shock. Because of steroids' anti-inflammatory properties, at the onset of the pandemic, synthetic steroids were widely used in the treatment of COVID-19.

In addition to the health crisis it caused, the virus became a political grenade. We heard it all, from conspiracy theories to hoax to "oh my God, what are we dealing with here?" At the onset of the chaos, a few political leaders called the virus a hoax. Jair Messias Bolsonaro, the president of Brazil, was one of them. It seems the virus didn't like that, as he got a nasty case of COVID-19 that was further complicated by a secondary fungal lung infection. I suspect steroids were in heavy play in his treatment, and I've heard other doctors speculate the same. The question is, did the steroids save his life? Maybe.

Failing in leadership, his country experienced one of the highest death rates globally. Bolsonaro, unfortunately, wasn't the only leader of a country to call COVID-19 a hoax as our own President of the USA, Donald Trump, and British Prime Minister Boris Johnson also did. Not leading by example, Trump went unmasked, rabble-rousing his followers, who did likewise. Not limiting contact exposure was a foolhardy thing to encourage, and we paid the price. Thanks to monoclonal antibody therapy, President Trump survived. Information that came later indicates the president was seriously sick with falling oxygen levels and infiltrates in his lungs, indicating pneumonia. He may well have been on his way to being placed on a respirator but was saved by modern American Medicine and some talented doctors. Trump said afterward, "Don't be afraid of it." And then he hid the fact that he'd received a vaccine before leaving the Whitehouse.

> *I could have written a prescription for myself for prednisone, as the burning sensation was constant and annoying, along with the continuous cough and feeling short of breath. Still, I chose to use a medicinal tincture of cannabis indica instead, which contains CBD. Unfortunately, at the time of my infection, I didn't have any CBD. Had I known that CBD would have been so effective in dialing down the chest inflammation, I would definitely have gotten some.*

> *I also noticed that the more refined carbohydrates I ate (honey in tea, maple syrup with pecans), the more my chest burned, and the more I coughed. I became dedicated to feeding myself right and limiting my refined carbohydrate intake as Coronavirus infections tend to flourish in people with elevated blood sugar.*

CHAPTER EIGHT

MAKING IT BETTER—THE SUN

HAVE A PROTRACTED CASE OF COVID-19?
You need to take a sunbath!
WANT TO AVOID IT? You need a sunbath!
TERRIBLY SICK? You need a sunbath!
LONG-HAULERS? You need a sunbath!

How does sunlight exposure fit into the picture of health? Well, that's simple. Health and vitamin D go hand in hand. Vitamin D's significant biological role is to maintain normal blood calcium levels and maintain strong bones. However, exposure to sunlight influences vitamin D production, affecting over 200 processes and influencing 1,000 gene expressions in the body. A deficiency in vitamin D is associated with thyroid disease, both hyperthyroidism and hypothyroidism and all else that's under the control of this master gland. Therefore, vitamin D protects and decreases the risk of osteoporosis, dental decay, hypertension, cancer, thinning hair, anxiety and the most common autoimmune diseases.

Our body follows a Circadian cycle, common to most living things. For humans, it's called the body's internal biological clock and regulates the sleep-wake cycle. We see patterns of all kinds of innate behaviors when birds fly south for the winter when penguins begin their courtship in March or April. When the Serengeti migration begins and ends. When plants bloom and fade, and all of this is regulated by time and the sun.

We, as higher species, are hunter-gatherers, not bat dwellers, on the computer or couch potatoes in front of the big screen. This means it's natural for us to be outside as the plants, trees, animals, insects, and birds to harness our energy. Like most living things, the sun is our energy source. One of vitamin D's jobs is to trigger the body's immune cells to produce antibodies, promoting a robust and essential immune system for a healthy life.

I was not surprised to have fallen sick at the end of winter. Due to months of less intense sunlight, vitamin D levels are lowest. If we followed hibernation laws, this might not be so bad, but we don't. We, humans, demand the same energy from our bodies year-round. An interesting observation is the birth-death cycle. It's natural that the human death rate goes up in December and January in the Northern Hemisphere and is lowest in July and August. Most babies are born in August, nine months after our "hibernation period," and fewer births occur in February, so it seems mother nature has a say in our entire existence from birth to death. Is there a correlation between birth rate and death rate and the solar cycle? In this heliotherapist's opinion, I say a resounding YES. We are, after all, just primates who like to break the laws of nature.

I most definitely consider myself a heliotherapist, so using sunlight as therapy is de rigueur. I believe sunbathing to be life-changing and lifesaving, and I believe COVID-19 recovery is helped by sun therapy. People of color are often adapted for tropical climates and are generally in the sun for extended periods, which is beneficial for vitamin D production. However, in temperate climates, depending on skin tone, they could need up to six times the amount of time in the sun to adequately synthesize a healthy vitamin D level and are at greater risk for vitamin D deficiency. Since vitamin D is associated with managing blood pressure and is often used, along with magnesium as an adjunct therapy for the treatment of hypertension, a lack of sufficient vitamin D levels may attribute to the higher levels of hypertension seen in African-Americans. Physicians need to be aware of this fact.

If indeed the virus can debilitate the body enough to kick it into hibernation mode by activating hormone rT3 Syndrome, don't you think sunlight exposure as one of the body's premier energy sources could be beneficial in routing you out of it? There is an absolute correlation between vitamin D deficiency and viral upper respiratory infections in medical literature, including COVID-19. Described as a complex multisystem disease, I remind you, upper respiratory infection is COVID-19's first presentation.

Being in the sun scares many people due to the propaganda machine's influence of sunscreen and sunglass companies. The 'Beast' ought to scare you more. As for the idea that sunlight ages you, it is the opposite. Of course, working outside for hours in the sunlight is not the idea here, especially if you are Caucasian. That will damage your skin, but moderate amounts of sunlight will improve your health and appearance, among many other important protections.

I am semi-retired and have the luxury of being in the sun at will, and I'm always without sunglasses. According to the ophthalmologist, my eyes had changes similar to those found in someone a decade younger. So, the idea that diffused sunlight damages your eyes is not accurate. How often do you see the oldest among us wearing shades? Almost never. YET, I caution that looking directly into the sun is not advised.

Concerning the argument, "You can just get vitamin D from your food and a pill." Any vitamin D is beneficial to the body, but going for artificial pills does not work as well as natural sunlight. When exposed to the sun, the synthesis of sun rays on the skin boosts nitric oxide production. Nitric oxide has the effect of dilation, not just of the small capillaries in the skin but also in arteries. Synthetic vitamin D does not offer protection from breast, colon, ovarian, leukemia, lymphoma, and prostate cancer, but natural sunlight does.

I cannot overemphasize this point enough; sunlight therapy is essential to a healthy body. Vitamin D protects against COVID-19 in two ways: (1). It boosts natural defenses and the antibodies against the virus, helping to avoid or lessen its severity if you get the virus; (2). It prevents exaggerated inflammatory responses to the disease.

A study by Medscape noted that severe vitamin D deficiency quadrupled the death rate of COVID-19 sufferers.[23] Patients with the lowest vitamin D levels were admitted to hospitals with the most severe infections and suffered the highest death rate. Not surprising since antibodies have a direct receptor for vitamin D to boost the immune system.

So, be sure to have adequate sunlight daily. I'm more than convinced to the point of being certain that Mother Nature has a hand in blessing us with the natural healing tools, diet, sleep, and sun, to help us co-exist with other living things on this earth—including opportunistic viruses.

I prescribe sun therapy to my patients to help them get over viral illness faster. Many have informed me that it's a New Mexican tradition for parents to place their sick children outside in the sun when they are sick, including during the winter. Amen, I say! Sun treatment is not a new idea for virus therapy. During the 1918 Spanish Flu pandemic, many photos show people lying on cots outside in the sun. It was recognized then that the people who insisted on being outside were recovering faster, so sunlight therapy became a treatment.

People look better with sunlight absorption because nitric oxide dilation flushes fluid from the face, and it looks sharper. The process of arterial dilations is a mechanism that also lowers heart attack rates. As the theory goes, a blood clot can keep moving past a plaque clogging up the heart's arteries that are dilated. You look better after sun therapy because you are better, and you feel great because you are healthier. One more thing about sunlight exposure, the libido gets a boost. Sunlight Research Forum in Veldhoven, Netherlands, had this to say, "Men who ensure their body is sufficiently supplied with vitamin D are doing good for their testosterone levels and their libido, among other things." The finding supports previous research that stated that an hour of sunshine could boost a man's testosterone level by up to 69 percent, and nitric oxide further increases the blood flow to the sex organs.[24]

The all-powerful vitamin D, if deficient, shows up in multiple ways. Patients often complain of fatigue, mood changes, migraines, hypertension, muscle cramps, bone pain, insomnia, and anxiety. Let me repeat; anxiety is a significant complaint among the sun phobic young. While it is clear that people do not die of vitamin D deficiency, they die due to diseases caused by vitamin D deficiency: heart disease, most common cancers, and now, COVID-19.

Let me urge you once again to get out into the sunlight as much as you can. Usually, if Caucasian, 20 minutes of daylight a day will keep vitamin D levels stable. If a person of color, depending on skin tone, you'll need an hour to an hour and a half in the sun. If you can't find sunlight for whatever reason, synthetic vitamin D pills are better than nothing, and I have certainly recommended them though I prefer the real deal; a life lived outside. If the next question you'd ask me after prescribing sun therapy is: What about skin cancer? My answer would be: I prefer skin cancer to the cancers mentioned above, attributed to low vitamin D.

Everything in the universe has a purpose, and the sun is no exception for life here on earth. Sunlight is our energy source. This pathway of human energy production allows us to become more active in summer and, as intended, to slow down during the winter or hibernation period, much like other living things.

As humans, we may be special, but we are members of the animal kingdom and cannot ignore the animal species' natural cycles. We do and introduce dis-ease in the body.

Sunbathing Protocol

The secret to successful sunbathing, which allows the body to naturally produce adequate vitamin D levels, is to expose more skin for short periods to direct sun rays. This will lessen the chance of skin damage and skin cancer. If the body produces adequate amounts of natural vitamin D levels during the summer months, vitamin D storage will increase to get the body through the winter during "hibernation."

During sunbathing sessions, put a cot in direct sunlight. Lie face down and absorb the rays for 15-20 minutes or one to one-and-a-half hours, depending on skin tone. Try to feel your body working, synthesizing vitamin D from sunlight into hormones. When done, place your hand on your lumbar area and then on the thigh. Notice the warmth on your back compared to the back of the thigh. The lumbar is the prizewinner for vitamin D production. This part of the body is the largest surface area meant to be exposed for hunter-gatherers bent over hunting and gathering. Since humans are designed to spend hours hunting and gathering in the summer to store for winter when the food source is scarce, what better way to capture rays. Frankly, I'm always amazed at the master plan of life.

Now turn over. In this position, while sunbathing, keep your face in the shade. For the appropriate time for your skin tone, aim for a moderate to deep tan. Keep your face out of direct sunlight as sun rays can damage the eyes if you look directly into it but under no circumstance should you wear sunglasses. The goal is to expose the entire body to the sun's healing rays, including the brain.

Because we are "hibernating" in the winter months, taking long walks during these dreary months will help keep the winter blues away and the concomitant winter weight gain under control.

> I sunbathed for hours from the first day of my illness until I was completely over the virus. I sunbathe year-round here in the desert. I just stayed out longer while sick. Contrary to popular advice, I sunbathe in the sunniest part of the

day for 15–20-minutes front and back. I haven't had a sunburn in 50 years. Luckily, I lived in a place where I could dedicate 30–40 minutes of sun therapy to help my immune system. Disease or no disease, I don't have time or inclination to be in the sun in the summer for longer than that. It's 100 degrees here, so it's in and out of 100-degree weather.

If you live in North America and can find ways to be outside, do it. Refracted sunlight coming into your eye is healthful in defeating seasonal associated depression syndrome (SADS). It also boosts concentration and makes it easier to fall asleep. You still may not get adequate vitamin D, but being outside is much preferable to being inside and taking vitamin D supplements. Vitamin D is essential for a healthy body. I want to share a few more facts and a story.

I'm constantly pushing myself to stay sharp. As I age, I do that both with diet and exercise. Before I arrived at my office at 9 a.m., I've eaten and have been out in the sunlight getting in a morning walk or run. Because of my acuity, I avoided a lawsuit because my mind was on point one morning, and I saw it coming a mile away. Unfortunately, frivolous lawsuits are the bane of a good doctor's existence, I being no exception. To make sure I add another component to my sharpness and sleep, you'll find me outside in the evening sun to stimulate melatonin production, making it easier to fall asleep.

I may wear my sunglasses at night for blocking intense artificial light!

Now for the facts. In 2018 CDC reported that worldwide, approximately a million and a half people died from Tuberculosis (T.B.) yet, that number in the US is under 10,000 because our public health service actively monitors people with T.B. [25] Until recently, two elderly doctors in Europe continued to treat children with tuberculosis infections of the bone in the Swiss mountains by having them sunbathe for hours. No medications were used. In New Mexico, there were sanatoriums in the mountains that treated people afflicted with T.B. because it was thought to be an ideal location altitude-wise. It was believed that the dry mountain air helped lung infections, but today we know that most of that help came from the sunlight's vitamin D production that activated the immune system.[26] This was no small feat, as tuberculosis is a mean, resistant, "I'm going to live in your body forever" bacterium, but it was still no match for the sun.

So, if sunlight bathing can help defeat T.B. and prevent cancer, why not allow it to work its magic on COVID-19? We know that sunlight can destroy coronavirus in the air. Give it a chance to destroy it in your body, and you're unlikely to be disappointed. Every one of your immune cells has a receptor for vitamin D; make sure to give them plenty of work by having plenty of vitamin D to attach to the antibody receptor. And it is free and natural! But if you have no sunlight, be ready to cough up (no pun intended $13-$20 a bottle) for synthetic vitamin D.

My final advice is that if you're out in the sun, have a healthy diet high in omega-3 and antioxidants to lessen skin damage. Astaxanthin, an antioxidant found in salmon, lobster and other shellfish, along with lycopene from tomatoes and beta carotene from carrots, all stop photoaging in rats and are often recommended by dermatologists as anti-aging foods. The sun causes significantly less skin aging if supported by an excellent diet. [27]

Conversely, a diet high in sugar and drinking alcohol will give you more wrinkles, whether you're in the sun or not. Sunbathing with a bad diet and daily alcohol intake? Yikes! More and more wrinkles.

It's time to inform skin propagandists to stop calling the sun the enemy.

CHAPTER NINE

MAKING IT BETTER
HYDROTHERAPY AND HEAT

Medical Hydrology, commonly referred to as hot springs bathing, thermal water therapy or mineral baths therapy, is the oldest continually applied medical treatment in Europe.[28] Physicians have been treating patients at thermal water spas for over 2,000 years. Under doctors' supervision, patients are treated in Central and South America, South Africa, Australia, and Asia with these healing therapies. The Spa-thermal water experience can last from one, two, three and up to six weeks, depending on the patient's condition. Many athletes utilize heat therapy in wet, dry, or infrared saunas to make them stronger and decrease pain from excessive muscle use.

The sweat lodge is an ancient ritual for purification and detoxification. In Asian countries, sauna bathing is a social ritual enjoyed by the entire family. In the United States, during the 1930s, bathing spas were also popular, with over 2,000 bathing establishments around the country. This holistic, therapeutic offering fell out of favor with American doctors for one reason or the other. That, however, was not because the treatment didn't work, but because this kind of therapy was not making enough money for the establishment. Doctors, dubbing its "curative ability" as useless, promoted its medical fall from grace. Yet, for much of the world, the 2,000 year-old treatment of medical hydrology continues.

During bathing in hot mineral water, the face and head are not affected by the heat, so ill and weak patients can tolerate this soothing, comfortable, and pleasurable therapy. European doctors have studied the physiological effects of thermal bathing extensively, and the following results have been observed:

Benefits of Hot Springs Bathing.
METABOLISM

- Especially important is the increased secretion of growth hormone (nicknamed the rejuvenator) released during hot springs bathing. This increases the cellular strength of muscles and aids cellular repair. Additionally, thyroid hormone levels rise and turn on the cell's energy packs, called mitochondria, increasing cellular activity for more efficient metabolism.

- Melatonin level increases and insomnia disappears.

- The adrenals produce anti-inflammatory hormones with prednisone-like qualities. Beta-endorphins, with their morphine-like attributes, are elevated. They act as the body's natural pain medication.

- Sex hormones increase in men and women, and libido is restored. The testosterone increase in men builds muscle mass, strength, and endurance. These hormones also have anti-aging properties.

BLOOD pH SHIFTS

Bathing in hot water causes blood pH to be more alkaline. Alkaline pH increases enzymatic and metabolic pathways, helping the body to operate more efficiently. It has often been said, a body with an alkaline pH is cancer-resistant.

DETOXIFICATION

When mineral water is hot enough, diaphoresis (sweating) occurs, and toxins such as arsenic, mercury and nicotine have been found in sweat droplets after bathing.

NERVOUS SYSTEM EFFECT

Heat therapy affects the neurologic system, both para and sympathetic. Parasympathetic tone increases (relaxation response), and sympathetic tone decreases. Serotonin levels increase, and anxiety and depression decrease. The mind goes into the meditative state, and the body relaxes. Hot springs bathing has been used historically for "Nervous Exhaustion."

IMMUNE RESPONSE

Hot mineral water bathing modulates immunity and activates the fever response. The body temporarily increases its temperature (1–3 degrees increases have been noted) and increases protective antibodies. This increase in antibody production may help rid the body of lingering viruses and bacteria. The rise in beta-endorphins also boosts the production of antibodies.

CIRCULATION EFFECT

There is documented evidence of an increase in the strength and contraction of the heart muscle. The arterial system dilates, and more blood flows to the skin. Small capillaries open with a greater exchange of oxygen, carbon dioxide and nutrients.

HYDROSTATIC PRESSURE

Pressure is exerted, and the upper and lower extremities can benefit from a decrease in swelling by a greater return of venous blood to the heart. The lymphatic system is affected by the greater movement of lymphatic fluids, which rids the body of waste products.

DIGESTION

Gastric secretions increase enhancing digestion and thereby enhancing the absorption of nutrients.

OBESITY AND WEIGHT LOSS

Due to the body's increase in hormones, there is a positive effect on decreasing appetite, and with a spa diet, better control of diabetes and weight loss has been observed.

ANTI-INFLAMMATORY

Due to various effects occurring simultaneously, from increased hormones, spa diet and solar therapy, there is a decrease in pain and inflammation, leading to better mobility of joints.

In the United States, medical errors such as anesthesia administration, hospital-acquired infections, missed or delayed diagnosis, avoidable delay in treatment, inadequate follow-up after treatment, inadequate monitoring after a procedure are the third leading causes of death after heart disease and cancer. The spa experience is extremely safe and life-enhancing. It is no wonder the medical establishment rejects the idea that mineral springs have any therapeutic value. I wonder why?

The true spa experience includes solar and hydrotherapy, a healthy diet, exercise and enhancing sleep aids such as CBD/THC. It is during sleep that most healing occurs, and this aids the body's ability to heal itself. In Truth or Consequences, we have an old saying regarding the medicinal effects of bathing: "Crawl In, Leap Out."

CHAPTER TEN

MAKING IT BETTER—SLEEP

If you're a dog owner, learn from your dogs. When they're sick with a virus, they have the good sense to lie down and sleep it off. So, did I. The body repairs itself during sleep, and you can be sure the big battle with the Coronavirus is taking place while you are in a sleep coma.

Always in the mornings, after a good sleep, I felt my best. The virus seemed to have regressed a bit, if only temporarily. After about an hour, I would again begin to feel poorly. Restlessness and my inability to fall asleep on the third night were the sickest I would feel. Seeing my oxygen level drop was scary, but cannabis indica took me out of the anxiety into a deep sleep. That morning of the fourth day, I started taking Chinese herbal medicine and hoped I'd be on my way to recovery. Indeed, everything was better, for an hour or so, and then, the misery, the cough, the burning and the shortness of breath resumed. As the illness progressed, I noticed that my symptoms would show up later and later in the day and increasingly after a good sleep.

Then one miraculous day, I didn't feel ill at all until the evening time. I knew I was on the road to recovery, but it would be another 48 hours until I turned the corner.

It was then that the feeling of being sick, the burning chest sensation, and the shortness of breath disappeared. My system had beaten the virus. The cough lessened significantly though it persisted for four weeks. The virus was not going down without a fight. The aftermath fatigue, however, lasted six weeks. COVID-19 just doesn't give up without a fight.

Again, I thank cannabis indica for the help with the cough and as the best sleeping medication for inducing deep sleep. A lack of sleep makes us more vulnerable to respiratory infections, and conversely, adequate sleep helps us defeat colds and the flu.

For me and many, getting a good night of sleep is a lifelong battle. Because I'm an insomniac, I could write a book giving good advice on sleeping on this topic of sleep. I've suffered for 20 years from insomnia, so imagine how happy I was to have discovered the influence of cannabis on sleep. I now sleep very well because of it.

Still, I have to play by the sleep rules, and I will share the essentials for sound sleep in this chapter.

The more you are outside in natural light (without sunglasses), the better you will sleep. Going out into the morning and afternoon sun sets the circadian rhythm and dramatically aids the brain in falling asleep. If you're sick, be outside, if possible, for as long as you can. If you're in a temperate climate, I'm not recommending you sit outside freezing, but I recommend that you find a place blocked from the wind to be outside—get a propane heater and be outdoors. Healing sunlight will improve sleep and get vitamin D topped off. If going outdoors is not possible, sit by an open window that allows direct sunlight on your skin.

Another important point, what one does all day affects the ability to sleep. It is wise to become acquainted with the many causes of insomnia so you can adjust your daily routine accordingly.

They are different forms of insomnia, and the remedies for each are different. The treatment chosen then should fit the particular cause of the sleep disruption. A lack of sleep resulting from not getting natural light or always wearing sunglasses causes a deficiency in the sleep hormone melatonin. A lack of sleep may occur from too much caffeine, overeating, eating late in the evening, being stressed out, being glued to the TV screen, or being exhausted from low adrenal and thyroid dysfunction. The list is long. So here it goes—forty-three factors that can disrupt sleep, and fortunately, most are under your control. When insomnia strikes, spend a little of your awake time roaming around in your mind to examine what might have happened that day to inhibit sleep.

SLEEP INHIBITORS

1. Alcohol. You might fall asleep, but that glass of wine will wake you up after a few hours.
2. Allergy medications.
3. Antidepressants.

4. Antihistamine can put you to sleep but then wake you up with frequent urination. In addition, they are associated with early-onset dementia.

5. Decongestants

6. Bright lights of the television or the computer screen, or any brightly lit environment can cause insomnia. If I go into a store in the evening, I wear sunglasses, also when watching the television at night. (Do it backward is one of my mottos, sunglasses at night and not during the day.)

7. Cigarettes. Nicotine is a stimulant, as are the toxins in tobacco.

8. Cold feet will prolong the time it takes to fall asleep for some crazy reason. The National Sleep Foundation recommends you warm your feet before sleeping. A heating pad is helpful and will reduce the time it takes to fall asleep

9. Decongestants.

10. Dehydration. Can you imagine? Not drinking enough water interferes with sleeping.

11. Depression.

12. Eating a big portion of meat for the evening meal can keep you awake. Eat meat at the earlier meal. I prefer to eat seafood for dinner.

13. Eating raw vegetables in the evening can disrupt sleep by causing you to get up a few times to urinate. Some vegetables and fruits have a pronounced diuretic effect, especially raw salad greens and watermelon. If you're

getting up to urinate more than twice, check what you've eaten, or you may have a urinary tract infection.

14. Eating sugar during the day can give you low blood sugar, up to12 hours later, and wake you from a sound sleep. When I wake up during the night and can't go back to sleep, I always check to see if I feel hungry. Unsweetened Hemp milk is my food of choice for the middle of the night snack.

15. Overeating, even healthy foods at evening meals, redirects blood flow needed for sleep to the gut to help in digesting the food consumed. If dinner is closer to bedtime for any reason, a few sardines in olive oil are a good choice for late eating as they are easily digestible and won't cause blood sugar problems. Eggs also are easily digested, and eating a diet rich in omega-3 apparently helps you sleep.

16. Eating too many carbohydrates for the evening meal can disturb sleep as it may cause low blood sugar.

17. Enlarged prostate and getting up to urinate frequently.

18. Exercising too late in the day can keep you awake.

19. Exhaustion from too much work and stress can lead to adrenals malfunction, which causes insomnia, usually early awakening.

20. Having heartburn will keep you awake.

21. High blood pressure medications.

22. Hyperthyroidism.

23. Hypothyroidism untreated or undertreated is associated with insomnia and sleep apnea.

24. Insomnia can be influenced by too many stimulants, caffeine, chocolate; working late into the evening; too much light stimulation.

25. Lack of exercise can cause insomnia

26. A lack of magnesium will keep you awake. Low magnesium can also cause restless legs syndrome, causing insomnia. Eating magnesium-rich foods and taking a magnesium supplement can cure these symptoms in some cases. Using magnesium skin spray and taking magnesium baths with Epsom salts, also known as magnesium sulfate, are other ways to get this trace element into your body. However, the biggest booster to absorbing magnesium is sunlight vitamin D exposure. Many people take Calms, an over-the-counter magnesium supplement that, when mixed with water, becomes an effervescent drink that promotes healthy magnesium levels and balances calcium intake. It helps you to feel less stressed and more relaxed at bedtime, helps muscle relaxation. A sign of being in a low magnesium state is twitching, especially around your eyes. If that happens, start your magnesium regimen, including sun therapy.

27. Lack of sexual activity will cause insomnia due to a lack of relaxation response.

28. Low vitamin D can interfere with sleeping and or taking vitamin D supplements too late in the evening. Your body metabolizes vitamin D and thinks it is daytime, with hours to go before it secretes melatonin, the sleep hormone.

29. Menopause and hot flashes, low estrogen, progesterone, and testosterone, are all associated with insomnia.

30. Moving around at night doing household chores is too stimulating—lower activity level a few hours before bedtime.

31. Noise.

32. Not enough thyroid medication or too much thyroid medication.

33. Deficiency of vitamin D, vitamin C and or deficiency or excess of Vitamin B12.

34. Obesity related to hypothyroidism can cause sleep apnea.

35. Pain.

36. Restaurant food depending on its quality, can keep you awake for a variety of reasons; over-eating, chemical overload of additives, taste enhancers, preservatives, and if not organic the pesticides, and fertilizers used in growing our food supply. Then there is the sodium load, which could have a negative effect on the renal and nervous systems, causing increased urination at night, not to mention a stimulating effect on the nervous system.

37. A room temperature of 68 degrees is perfect since sleep occurs during the coolest part of the 24-hour day.

38. Snoring from a bed partner.

39. Spices especially (listen up), black pepper. Prepared foods from health stores always seem to have pepper—and forget about having Mexican food at night.

40. ADD and ADHD medications, Ritalin and Adderall

41. Stress, Stress, Stress.

42. The chemicals in junk food; processed food is full of chemicals. In particular, MSG is a stimulant and can cause insomnia. Sad too, because who doesn't love MSG-drenched Chinese food?

43. A deficiency of Melatonin, the sleep hormone easily remedied by taking Melatonin at bedtime.

I do not follow the advice to get out of bed if unable to sleep to do some low-level activity. Preferably lie in bed, in the darkness, and evaluate your day. Try calming yourself with a little meditation. Regarding a hangover from taking a little extra cannabis and CBD on sleepless nights, I feel this is better to have a cannabis hangover than sleep-deprived, especially when sick. Being sleep-deprived is bad for health in every way and cognitively increases the risk of making mistakes, having an accident, or having a heart attack or stroke. A cannabis hangover is less dangerous.

Quick Do and Don'ts Tips

A little sun tip that is beneficial to help sleep earlier in the evening. Go outside without sunglasses as soon as you awake. Stay out for at least 20 minutes. Do it again as the sun sets. This signals the brain to secrete Melatonin, the sleep hormone. Make it a habit and notice how sleep rituals change. You'll be sleeping at the hour that is healthiest for you.

1. Do exercise in the morning or afternoon.

2. Don't exercise at night. It will increase endorphins, a no-no for sleep

3. Do learn about the acupressure points that are associated with inducing sleepiness. You can find helpful videos about this on YouTube.

4. Don't keep distractions in the bedroom, such as cell phones and tablets.

5. Do add a fern to the bedroom...it gives off oxygen and absorbs carbon dioxide.

6. In the evening, don't watch TV or stare at a computer screen, and if you do, wear sunglasses. I do.

7. Do keep your room temperature at about 68 degrees

8. Do develop a meditation practice

Don't forget the body is in healing mode while you sleep, so sleep maximally.

CHAPTER ELEVEN

MAKING IT BETTER— CHINESE HERBAL MEDICATIONS TO THE RESCUE

A doctor friend informed me that the 3,000 year-old tradition of medicine in China has nothing in common with the almost 200-year-old practice of western medicine in the USA. Not a single thing. Though a well-known fact in health circles that the Chinese are healthier than the Americans, I was clueless. That was an enlightening moment in this young doctor's career and piqued my interest.

The use of Traditional Chinese Medicine (TCM) is far more widespread in Asia and Africa [29] than in Western societies and addresses just about every discomfort and disease the body may experience. WHO estimates that up to 80 percent of the populations of Asia and Africa use herbal medicine.[30] These herbs enhance the body's healing abilities with little to no side effects! The baffling thing is that many synthesized drugs are derivatives of naturally occurring herbs and plants trying to mimic their effect. Prescription drugs such as digitalis, which come from the foxglove plant, also aspirin and quinine are Pharmaceutical medications from plant derivatives currently used to treat Parkinson's, COPD, Malaria, Alzheimer's, and Cholesterol lowing medications.

Why then not just use the real deal? The answer is supply and demand. We can make a lot more stuff in the lab than nature can provide.

As I hope you know by now, many confluences, diet, stress levels, lack of rest, value systems, environment, etc., contribute to one's overall health. What we do not need to add are the side effects of many drugs that read like a laundry list of debilitations. As a holistic doctor, I've always been interested in Traditional Chinese Medicine (TCM). It is far more in harmony with my belief in natural healing. I became even more convinced when COVID-19 struck.

The virus was first identified in China in December 2019, but by March of 2020, infection rates there had dropped to single-digit numbers while the numbers skyrocketed worldwide. What was going on here? A NIH.GOV study showed that the Chinese government mandated that TCM be used on highly infectious and pernicious viruses as well as conventional medicine. The study concluded that TCM was effective in preventing COVID-19 and that China's citizens' high level of compliance and immediate lockdown were significant factors in controlling the disease. Indeed, 90 percent of the Chinese population took TCM, and the containment of the virus was also well-managed as all the citizens wore masks. It was further noted that medical staff could prevent iatrogenic diseases introduced in a hospital setting during treatment, such as cross-contamination of pathogens infections. Using TCM therapy and following protocols of mask-up effectively managed these risks. I later became interested in learning how TCM could help contain my COVID-19.

TCM has a well-documented history of treating infectious diseases. At the height of the Italian spike in infection, China sent 100,000 boxes of anti-COVID-19 herbal medications to Italy. It appeared to have had a dramatic effect on managing the infection.[31] China also sent herbal medicines to France, Canada, Iraq, and Korea, and they too had success in lowering COVID-19 cases. Since then, the demand for TCM has skyrocketed worldwide, and Asia continues to do an admirable job of decreasing the severity of the illness and managing the virus.

Natural Remedies Have their Basis in Science, too.

In 2005, I overheard a woman tell the following story in a café in Salzburg. She'd had hand surgery for a Dupuytren Contracture, a condition that caused one or more of her fingers to stay stuck in a flexed position. Two days after surgery in a Paris hospital, her hand blew up with an infection. She was administered every antibiotic known to man without improvement. When the doctors recommended amputation, she said, "Merde, non!" and left the hospital. She consulted a Chinese Medicine doctor who told her to continually drink a tablespoon of vinegar in water for three days. Within the first 24 hours, her hand had returned to its normal size. So, what gives?

Here it was, a bacterial infection resistant to broad-spectrum antibiotics was successfully treated with a household item that had zero side effects or cost. I was glad to hear this story.

An old German remedy for strep throat is sucking on cloves of raw garlic. Garlic has such powerful antibacterial properties that the Group-A Streptococcus bacteria, causing tonsillitis, dies and infections in the tonsils resolve with the use of garlic. Garlic also has anti-viral properties. Many of nature's herbs developed and perfected over centuries have been used in Chinese medicine. I'd had enough treatment success with TCM for my patients' aliments to try it with my COVID-19 infection. And I did with success. So, if there is value in adding this alternative medical approach to COVID-19 treatment to aid in recovery, do it!

Here is what to do. Go to a Chinese herbal doctor. He or she will put you on traditional Chinese herbal medication that has been proven to stop bacterial and viral infections. If you go to a medical provider for a COVID-19 infection, there's a good chance they'll put you on a Z-Pak and steroids. This should be the last resort. If you have a wet cough full of infected phlegm, then I agree Z-pak could make sense, but if the cough remains dry, it's unlikely you have a secondary infection, so a drug that treats bacterial infections will not work on viral infections. Skip the antibiotic and its side effects of destroying good bacteria.

In 2021, in the US, Z-pak (azithromycin) was listed as the third most often prescribed medication pushing synthetic thyroid replacement, Synthroid, i.e., levothyroxine to number four. As an aside and entirely off-topic, but based on these stats, I've spent some time wondering if antibiotics are the culprits behind obesity and autoimmune diseases. Antibiotics destroy good gut bacteria. The destruction of good gut bacteria decreases digestion, impeding the breakdown of food to release the needed nutrients from protein, carbohydrates, fats, vitamins, and minerals. Nutritional deficiency leads to overeating to compensate for missing nutrients. So, could it be that partially digested food moving through the bloodstream is seen by the body as a foreign substance and riles up the immune system to attack?

If inadequately digesting food is a problem, antibiotics are certainly not what's needed when you're sick. Before taking antibiotics, ask the provider if they are absolutely necessary.

> *My first step on the first day I knew I was sick was to fill large gelatin capsules (found in health stores) with garlic powder, ginger powder and cayenne powder. I took it with three capsules of dehydrated vinegar three times a day. After three days without improving, my partner reminded me to try the Chinese medicine herbs, which had been gifted to us by Jim English, the owner of the company, Tango Nutrition. It's a product called ImmunoPhase®, an improved version of a powerful herbal immune support formula developed by a master traditional Chinese medicinal herb doctor in 2003, specifically the SARS outbreak in Hong Kong. I didn't think to take the herbals sooner because my brain, sick with this virus, wasn't thinking. I immediately started taking TCM on the morning of my fourth day of deep malaise, cough, and fever. Forty-eight hours later, on the morning of the sixth day, I woke symptom-free for most of the day, only to relapse and battle the Beast for yet another week. It took an additional two weeks of coughing and laying around before it was all over.*

The TCM I took, as I said, was ImmunoPhase®. It's made up of the following ingredients—Isatis root, Kutdu, Pubescent Holly Root, European Verlain Root. Chinese Wormwood, Sichuan Lovage root, Magnolia Flower, Shielf Fern Herb, Honeysuckle Flower, Forsythia Fruit Siberian Cockburn, Fruit

Fragrant Angelica, Gypsum Fibrosum Notopterygium Root, and Bupleurum Root.

Before popping synthetic drugs into the body with myriad side effects, consider visiting a Chinese medical doctor or have a telephone conversation with one.

CHAPTER TWELVE

MAKING IT BETTER OR MAKING IT WORSE—HYDROXYCHLOROQUINE, Z-PAK, AND REMDESIVIR

In 2013, the FDA issued a warning that Z-Pak (taken in the US like eating M&M's) can cause a fatal ventricular arrhythmia called Torsade de Pointes.[32] Unfortunately, Hydroxychloroquine, an immunosuppressant and antimalarial drug bandied about as a drug cure for COVID-19, was also a misstep and might have led to a bad outcome for patients. Combining these two drugs in COVID-19 treatment is questionable, particularly in an elderly patient with multiple illnesses. Z-Pak, in conjunction with Hydroxychloroquine, increases the risk of sudden cardiac death. This is especially concerning if levels of magnesium and potassium, common in the infirm and elderly, are low.

If a patient has cardiovascular disease, Hydroxychloroquine by itself increases the risk of the same arrhythmia caused by Z-Pak. Clearly, these drug choices cannot be good options for people with serious health issues, especially cardiovascular disease.

A doctor I highly respect believes the combination of drugs can work but stresses that it must be started early. However, this regimen failed him as he became ill with COVID-19. I have no recommendations except to say I wouldn't take or prescribe them. When patients have requested it, I've said no. Why? Because first, one needs to be pretty healthy to take this combination of drugs, and their effectiveness against the virus is speculative. I suspect that hydroxychloroquine's loudest supporters, Bolsonaro and Trump, took it prophylactically, yet they got sick anyway. Even the doctor who recommended it got COVID-19. The markedly heightened risk of a bad outcome for really sick people and maybe not-so-sick people gives me pause in making such recommendations.

After taking Z-Pak, I had a doctor friend who developed Torsade's de Pointes, which is resistant to treatment and is usually fatal. He put up a brave fight in the critical care unit, going in and out of this ventricular arrhythmia until he stayed in it, flatlined, and his heart stopped.

The next drug used for treating COVID-19 is Remdesivir. An RNA-inhibitor, Remdesivir, is an antiviral drug and was used to treat SARS-CoV-1. At the onset of the COVID-19 pandemic, there was no data on its effectiveness in treating this novel coronavirus. The World Health Organization (WHO) recommended against its use because it did not improve the death rate.[33] Shortly after that, an article published in the New England Journal of Medicine (NEJM) said giving Remdesivir could shorten the disease's duration and get patients off oxygen sooner.[34] Within days, Remdesivir was authorized for COVID-19 use. It is antiviral, and I agree it was worth a try, but whether or not it works, it was not going to be handed out like the anti-flu medication Tamiflu. Remdesivir is a series of injections given daily for five days, usually for severely ill hospitalized patients and carries a cost of $3,100.

The consensus in the medical community, I believe, was; if one was going to succumb to COVID-19, this medication could not keep them alive. If they were going to survive, the drug would speed up recovery, and patients could be discharged from the hospital. And if you recall, hospital beds were like gold.

Since the onset of the "Beast," several vaccines have hit the market, and scientists are working on an antiviral medication for COVID-19 to be prescribed much like Tamiflu for the flu. Oral antiviral drugs have successfully been developed for HIV, Hepatitis, Herpes, Simplex-Shingles, and the Flu. Pfizer claims to have developed a medication in pill form that can be taken at home for COVID-19.[35]

Hopefully, this medication, a protease inhibitor, will be our ticket out of this catastrophic illness and help the unvaccinated as we head into the new Delta variant storm.

CHAPTER THIRTEEN

MAKING IT WORSE—SUGAR

The novel COVID-19 is, apparently, a sugar addict. There are stories of patients going into hypoglycemia (low blood sugar) arriving at the emergency room with glucose levels of 30 or 40 mmol/L.Vs. (normal levels are 140 or less mmol/L). We know this virus loves obese and diabetic people with high glucose levels in their blood. It may seem counterintuitive to starve such a monster of carbohydrates, but if you're giving in to the sugar craving that comes with most viral infections, particularly this one, my best advice is to "Starve the 'Beast' of Sugar."

It should be noted that the anatomical part of the coronavirus, which does the invading, has spikes proteins covered in glucose. Does this mean the novel coronavirus uses glucose to invade a cell? It sounds like it could indeed be the case.

Eating sugar and fructose has long been associated with bad health and with getting colds, flus and cancer. After eating sugar, it seems the immune system temporarily crashes, and the tiredness that follows a sugar binge is in the immune cells taking a rest.[36] When the immune system is on pause, a pernicious virus has the advantage of getting a foothold in cells. Since viruses may invade seeking a world with an excellent glucose supply, we want to prevent that.

Sugar is an elixir for any virus and bacteria. Excess sugar in your system permits the virus to propagate in an already COVID-19 compromised system. I stress being an educated patient, so you have the power and the knowledge to make choices. I heard of an obese woman who'd contracted the virus. She was on a ventilator for days, and the moment she came off the ventilator, she couldn't wait to have her favorite drink, a cherry Coke! Was drinking sugar-laden Coke feeding her coronavirus invasion into a super invasion all along? Most likely. A diet laden with junk food may be one of the tickets to being placed on a ventilator if you contract COVID-19. It's called junk food because there is little nutritional value even if it tastes "good." Lay off the stuff not only for the sake of COVID-19 but permanently for optimum health.

In the United States, we have numerous sugar festivals to induct children into a life of sugar addiction. Valentine's Day, Easter, Memorial Day, the Fourth of July, Labor Day, Halloween, Thanksgiving, Christmas, and New Year's. All are celebrated by eating sweets. Small amounts of the addictive substance, a cookie here, a candy bar there keeps the craving going, is literally feeding the addiction. If you are addicted to caffeinated soft drinks, I'm sorry to say that you're an uninformed consumer who the junk food industry has captured.

Please understand these legal drugs that are so easy to get at the supermarket are indeed another beast. The reality is that sugar is as addictive as cocaine, activating the same pleasure centers in the brain. I've heard it said that one could use cocaine eight times before being hooked. Consume sugar just once, and you're addicted. Maybe this is an over-exaggeration, but all of us know that consuming sugar is terrible for us. That we cannot stop eating it is the intent of the food industry consumer marketers. Most of us who are sugar addicts go through withdrawal when we stop. Like any addiction, we can try to go without it, but if we fall off the wagon and have some sugar, most will be hooked again. If you're a sugar addict like I am, you'll have to battle it for an entire lifetime or succumb to it. While in the abstinence period, it does get easier with time until you don't crave it at all, so find the strength "just to say no" and get yourself free of this addiction.

Known health conditions that sugar causes are dental decay, obesity, diabetes, low blood sugar, fatigue, irritability, less efficient liver functions, brain inflammation, and cancer. In a laboratory rat experiment, fructose, the sweetener in soft drinks, was also shown to interfere with vitamin D absorption. I can't see why it would be different in humans.

And let me not get started on how it impacts workdays. Getting tired after consuming sugar is common, making your job more challenging due to sugar-induced fatigue. What a deal! Huh?

So, people with COVID-19 who are craving sugar, fructose and corn syrup should stop eating it now! If not, it's going to be the battle of a sugar addict, the coronavirus, and you. I wonder who wins?

I now have no choice but to confess that I was eating sugar when I contracted the virus, although minimally. I hadn't gone through sugar withdrawal after Christmas and had stayed hooked on Belgian Chocolate. I'd also been eating sugar when I got sick with the flu in 2008, another Christmas Day and after a sugar binge. It took contracting COVID-19 to force me to cut it out. I had little appetite anyway, so it wasn't too difficult to cool it with the chocolate. But there were days, even during my illness, when the sugar cravings were overwhelming. I decided to stop the cravings by using a little honey and maple syrup one morning. Within a few hours, it seemed to have aggravated the infection, almost like a relapse, and my symptoms worsened: more cough, more chest burning sensation, shortness of breath, and it felt like the infection was worsening. I imagined the coronavirus having a field day saying, "Hey, keep it up. We can hang here, lots of glucose to fuel our lives."

So, I cut it out. Really.

CHAPTER FOURTEEN

MAKING IT WORSE —ALCOHOL

Not surprisingly, alcohol consumption is associated with an increased risk of upper respiratory infections—WHO advises against drinking to avoid COVID-19.[37] I'll go along with that. The alcohol industry has blatantly lied to us, giving the erroneous impression that a drink a day for women and two drinks for men was safe and may even benefit cardiac health! To me, it's just another more money, more money scheme.

From the American Cancer Society's point of view, "Drinking alcohol raises the risk of some cancers: cancers of the mouth, throat, larynx, esophagus, colon and rectum and breast cancer in women.[38] The less alcohol you drink, the lower the risk."

I vote no on alcohol. WHO also states alcohol will make your COVID-19 infection worse.[39] Don't forget some alcohol, such as sweet wines, can be laden with sugar. When I hear of people drinking a 6-pack per night or taking two shots daily or see their shopping carts with bottles of alcohol concoctions and beer (so fattening and carbohydrate-rich), I can hardly believe there are people who think that this is a natural way to go through life. Everyone consuming alcohol regularly or binge drinking ought to, in my cannabis consulting opinion, consider a change to cannabis. No amount of alcohol is healthful.

A woman I worked with used to binge drink on weekends, five drinks on Saturday night, and then deal with a hangover on Sunday. Since using a gummy of cannabis, she has cut down to two drinks, which is a big improvement. More than one of my patients returning for yearly cannabis renewal cards tell me they've stopped drinking, and according to one patient, a fifth daily.

If you are jonesin' for alcohol and you have a COVID-19 infection, cannabis will soften the withdrawal. I'm well aware that withdrawal from alcohol is challenging in the extreme and potentially dangerous, so seek your doctor's and support groups' help. It is quite a feat and a real accomplishment. You have my sympathy.

Unfortunately, alcohol consumption is up since the COVID-19 pandemic overtook our lives, and that's sad. It's a double whammy against our health. If you remember, alcohol interferes with sleep, while cannabis indica is the excellent sleep aid of all time. Mixing cannabis and alcohol is absolutely not recommended. Peace out, my friend, smoke a joint, and forget the booze.

CHAPTER FIFTEEN

MAKING IT WORSE—STOP FEEDING LOUSY FOODS TO YOUR IMMUNE SYSTEM

Good health begins with the foods we consume. By now, you've had an appreciation and some understanding of the body's complex integration and interdependent systems and processes. Every day the body is working hard to keep us healthy, and we can help it by the foods we feed it. As the building blocks of health, foods are the starting point of great health and keeps the body in homeostasis. With the threat of the virus, it's an excellent time to revisit daily eating habits. If you haven't already, how about starting a nourishing diet now? Focus all the body's energy on immune energy-building foods and avoid having your energy zapped trying to digest the lasagnas you just ate.

From the last couple of chapters, you know that sugar and alcohol are part of the bad foods we put in our body that burden the immune system. In COVID-19 and Post-COVID Syndrome, the already overburdened immune system needs all the support it can get from a superior diet. A good diet will give the immune system a break from foods associated with an autoimmune attack. Another thing to be aware of is that the same group of antibodies, the B cells that attack COVID-19, are involved in the pathogenic immune response in food allergic enteropathy. Skip and avoid foods known to rile the immune system or those associated with an auto-immune disease. Which foods?

Stay clear of any foods with gluten, dairy and eggs. Avoid pizza, bread, cookies, ice cream, cheese, nachos, pretzels, and forget about other refined carbohydrates like rice, corn, fruit, etc. If you have the virus or Long COVID Syndrome, commit to not eating flour products, eggs and dairy products in particular, even if non-hormone fed.

Eat the stuff of the cavemen who ate directly from the source. *The Autoimmune Solution* by Amy Myers, M.D. has an excellent diet to kick start your new lifestyle. Eating clean during your illness will keep your strength up and reduce inflammation in your body. Go practically paleo—no grains, no sugar, no fruit, and limit certain vegetables. Instead, eat meat, fish, seafood, nuts, sweet potatoes and a few other vegetables. More about foods in chapter twenty-one.

CHAPTER SIXTEEN

MAKING IT WORSE—DEHYDRATION

Next to the sun, water is your friend. Ninety-five percent of the body's cells are made up of water and for a good reason. Viral infections cause dehydration, and with them, there is increased fluid loss due to fevers, an activated immune system and a suppressed appetite. Be aware of the need to replenish water during an illness. I know drinking water has been bantered about as a positive health tip, but everything should always be in moderation. Do not be misled by the 'more is better' theory. If you drink too much water, you're washing out essential minerals, which is the last thing you want to do.

For most adults and until the 1970s, we can safely drink eight glasses of water a day. If still thirsty, drink more, particularly if you have a fever. If urine becomes clear, not its usual straw color, you've consumed too much water. If it is too yellow, you're dehydrating and will need to drink more water until it becomes its usual straw-yellow color.

Here's some good advice I follow. Because we tend to be most dehydrated in the mornings, upon rising and during the first hour, drink two glasses or 16 oz of water. Within two to three hours, drink two more 8 oz glasses, and you are halfway there. During the afternoon to early evening, drink the other four glasses of water. Try not to drink water with food. This thins out the gastric acid required to digest food efficiently, so drink water on an empty stomach.

If you can tolerate it, add a little vinegar to the water. It is considered a digestive aid, among its many other benefits. I take vinegar in capsule form because I'm a weakling and do not like the taste of the stuff, but I'm a firm believer in its positive effect on health. It seems ancient civilizations knew this too. While ruling the ancient world, the Romans carted barrels of vinegar to drink during war expeditions because of the health benefits it affords the body.[40]

I have read that Long Haulers complain of dramatic thirst. Drinking way too much water puts them at risk for low sodium, i.e., hyponatremia, low magnesium and potassium, which increase the risk for cardiac arrhythmias and muscle cramping. The cause of the excessive thirst is hormonal, a defect in antidiuretic hormone secretion caused by the illness. If you find yourself thirsty after excessive water drinking, my advice would be to bring water consumption back to normal; let's say to ten glasses over twenty-four hours, then nine glasses, and then back to eight glasses.

CHAPTER SEVENTEEN

MAKING IT WORSE—VEGETARIANISM AND VEGANISM

Everything needed to optimize the body's antibody production is low or missing in a vegetarian or vegan diet. According to a Harvard study, evidence suggests that deficiencies in zinc, selenium, iron, copper, folic acid vitamins A, B6, C, and E alter the immune response in animals.[41] (Typically, vegetarians and vegans may already be deficient in omega 3, zinc, selenium, iron, vitamin B12, omega-3 and vitamin D.) No one should think that taking supplements signifies an improvement over getting nutrients naturally in the diet. The vegetarian diet also relies on eggs, dairy, and grains, which can negatively affect the immune system and, you now know, are associated with auto-immune illnesses.

Let me argue the myth that vegetarians are healthier and live longer in one or two sentences. Vegetarians are health nuts and can outlive the carnivore eating processed meat, junk foods and consuming alcohol. But compare a health nut vegetarian with a health nut omnivore, and the statistics change. In addition, the carnivore has more muscle, which is an advantage in an aging human. There are, of course, arguments and studies on both sides.

A couple of hundred years ago, the city of Graz in Austria had a very high infant mortality rate, and the queen wanted to know why. At the decree of Queen Maria Theresa of Austria, they began performing autopsies on all the citizens of the town who died.

The great American thyroid doctor, Broda Barnes M.D., spent 20 summers in Graz with American medical students reviewing 70,000 pathology reports. They discovered the increased mortality was linked to iodine deficiency. Iodine deficiency leads to Hypothyroidism. The body cannot make thyroid hormone without iodine because the thyroid hormone itself is a clump of iodine.[42] Remember, the thyroid is a master gland that influences all body systems—an incidental finding by Dr. Barnes: there was an increased death rate among vegetarians for any cause.

It's hard to tell vegetarians this. They are a pretty tough lot. More than a few have roughed me up when they come into urgent care frustrated because they can't shake the virus that's been dragging them down for weeks. When I ask the question, how much red meat do you eat, and they say none. I'm vegetarian; I advise them that the vegetarian diet is deficient in the nutrients the immune system needs. That's when they become irate and want to knock my block off. Sometimes, they will inform me that I'm ignorant and a quack and demand to see a different provider. That's when I tell them, "You make your muscle out of broccoli and tofu, and I'll make mine out of elk meat," and run out of the door. No one should think the life of a truth-telling doctor is easy.

CHAPTER EIGHTEEN

MAKING IT BETTER—TRY THE PALEO DIET

Paying particular attention to food intake is even more important if you have the virus. Going the natural way in eating habits is ideal for the immune system.

B and T cells, specific antibodies produced by the body to combat COVID-19, have receptors for vitamin D, vitamin B12 and thyroid T3. The mitochondria, the cell's energy factory, need magnesium to run, and omega 3 is required to form new cell membranes. Omega 3 deficiencies negatively impact immune function, but before going overboard on fish oil pills, understand that too much omega 3 also has a negative effect. It can cause elevated blood sugar, bleeding, stroke, low blood pressure and vitamin A toxicity.

As the norm, my holistic patients are encouraged to eat a low glycemic diet, emphasizing omega 3 and vitamin B12 and B6 rich foods. So too, should patients with COVID-19 get on a paleo diet, as suggested in a previous chapter. Choose grass-fed butter, fatty cuts of grass-fed beef, lamb, Alaskan or Pacific salmon and affordable sardines in olive oil. The double-layer means you'll eat sixteen little fish instead of three larger ones. I'm all for eating wild game, which is one of the benefits of living in New Mexico: we have access to elk, venison, bison, oryx and antelope.

I recommend eating foods high in fat that convert to omega 3: nuts, seeds, avocados, olives, olive oil, coconut and coconut oil. Avoid dairy except for grass-fed butter. Choose other sources of probiotics besides yogurts, such as kombucha and fermented vegetables. I avoid eating chicken because it is linked to weight gain, but organic noodle-less chicken soup may be irresistible at this time. Try mung bean noodles instead if you have to have noodles. It may be strange to say this, but people who eat chicken put on more weight than those who avoid it. Go figure, and if you don't believe me, research it.

Avoid whole and refined grains, including flour, rice, and corn. They all convert to glucose. Especially skip flour, all types and oatmeal unless it is non-gluten oatmeal. If you must, quinoa is the preferred choice. Limit the carbohydrates you feed the 'Beast' and opt for resistant starch foods such as potatoes, sweet potatoes, plantains, taro, and yucca. What is it about starch? Starch doesn't digest.

These tubers are referred to as prebiotics because they are food for the good bacteria in the gut. They are delicious, and some are hard to find, so try ethnic stores. Just cook them like potatoes, but not before peeling them. Buy mung bean starch noodles and sweet potato noodles in the regular grocery store, but you might find they are less expensive in an Asian market.

Eat low glycemic vegetables, asparagus, lettuce, garlic, especially onions and high in vitamin A vegetables like carrots and sweet potatoes. While ill, skip the vegetables that are thyroid hormone blockers, such as broccoli, kale, and other cruciferous vegetables. They will interfere with thyroid production and can cause low thyroid function. For people with thyroid disease, they should be skipped period, COVID or no COVID. Also, skip the nightshade family of vegetables, tomatoes, eggplant, peppers, and limit potatoes. These foods are associated with inflammation.

Forget about sugar and fructose. Limit fruit to one a day or better still; avoid them altogether. Avoid mangoes, bananas, dates, and pineapple due to their high glycemic content. An exception here is apple peel which is so healthful for us. Daily I eat an apple by eating the peel only. Avoid vegetable oils such as canola, margarine, corn, safflower, and soy oil. Avoid prepared deli meats.

Cook meat and fish slowly at low heat. Eat foods that make the thyroid stronger since thyroid hormone does the heavy lifting of energy production. Eat fish, shellfish, and seaweed. Crispy wakame wrappers made with olive oil are a good choice.

An article in the New York Times blog "EMBRACING LOW CARB-HIGH FAT" suggests that following a paleo diet will lower cholesterol and cardiovascular risks and increase muscle mass. Great. Please listen.[43]

CHAPTER NINETEEN

MAKING IT BETTER—SUPPLEMENTS, VITAMIN, MINERAL AND NUTRACEUTICAL THERAPY

Always, as you might glean, I recommend sun therapy and natural diets to get the required trace elements and supplements the body needs to stay healthy. If for any reason getting these nutrients naturally is not possible, it's best to go on nutrimental therapy rather than to be without the essential trace elements the body needs.

There are fourteen trace elements your body needs for optimization, some of which are iron, copper, zinc, selenium and manganese. These elements are required for many of the body's physiological and biochemical processes. Fortunately, the trace elements are found in red meat, concentrated in organ meats, and most of them are also found in fish and shellfish.

Necessary Vitamins and minerals for a healthy body.

- The single most important thing to do is take the two wonder supplements: vitamin D and Magnesium Citrate or glycinate 400 mgs. Take one to two with food, dividing the dose according to meals. Magnesium helps activate vitamin D. Additionally, the enzymes that metabolize vitamin D require magnesium as a cofactor for enzymatic functions in the liver and kidneys. Try and take as many as four a day if possible. Consider a magnesium boost— Epsom salt bath. Fill the bathtub with hot water, let it sit for 10 minutes to warm the tub, empty, and refill with hot water. Now, add two cups of Epsom salts and soak away. The tub will stay warmer longer. Also, explore the possibility of magnesium spray therapy, not expensive and found in the health store. In addition, eat magnesium-rich foods–semi-dark/dark and coconut sugar or Stevia sweetened, chocolate, pumpkin seeds, sunflower seeds, and greens.

- Vitamin C 1000-2000 mgs daily divided with meals. During an active infection, increases vitamin C levels to 3000 mgs daily.

- If hypothyroid, take Kelp 225 mcg daily with the main meal. If not hypothyroid, take anyway, another wonder supplement. This is the essential supplement for thyroid production since iodine is the thyroid hormone's building block (if hyperthyroid, <u>do not</u> take Kelp). Note iodine is the original supplement. Since 1924 it was added to salt to prevent hypothyroidism.

- Omega 3, take 1–2 capsules daily (natural sources: Alaska salmon). No more than 3,000 mg per day.

- Vitamin B12 1000 mcg sublingual (under the tongue) every day. Double the dose in an infection.

- Potassium 100 mgs and twice daily with food.

- Virgin Coconut Oil. Dr. Bronner's is a good one
- Extra Virgin Olive Oil (California Ranch is pure olive oil)
- Extra Virgin Avocado Oil
- Hemp Oil

How many tablespoons of oil daily? At least three.

- Avocado or olive oil–based mayonnaises
- Butter from grass-fed cows is a good source of omega 3. Eat without cooking it. Butter does not contain the trouble-making milk proteins
- Eating fat doesn't cause weight gain. On the contrary, it helps with weight loss by satiating appetite. It is carbohydrates that cause you to gain weight.

Take all supplements with food. Double up on the dose during illness, particularly if you're a vegetarian or older than fifty.

I want to make a note here about vitamin D deficiency. It is not unusual to find that vitamin D dosage recommendations are all over the map, depending on who you ask. If vitamin D is deficient, it is best to get advice from a doctor. Before starting a regime, get a baseline vitamin D level to determine the body's needs. Two thousand international units (IU) daily with magnesium is conservative and what I recommend to my younger patients for normal supplement replacement. Vitamin D 4000 IU daily is what I recommend if the patient is sick and in their 60's or 70's. If a patient is ill with COVID-19 or Long COVID Syndrome, I suggest checking vitamin D levels every eight weeks after therapy begins.

In general, these IUs are pretty good benchmarks, but depending on other factors such as weight, obesity, and hypothyroidism, more or less may be recommended. Pay attention to recommended levels because too much vitamin D can create vitamin D toxicity, leading to a buildup of calcium, which causes its own set of issues for the body. Doses of 10,000 IU daily, in my opinion, may be excessive. However, it has been deemed safe by the Endocrine society. There is controversy around this as the Institute of Medicine and WHO has put the daily upper limit for vitamin D supplementation at 4000 IU for COVID-19 patients and adults in general. If taking vitamin D, always, one other highlight: always supplement magnesium with it or be at risk for a magnesium deficiency.

CHAPTER TWENTY

MAKING IT BETTER—KOMBUCHA, FERMENTED VEGETABLES, PROBIOTICS

Pay some attention to gut bacteria. Good gut bacteria help with overall health and gives a sense of psychological well-being; strange but true. The reason there's so much noise about probiotics is that they're ultra-important. There is even speculation that altered gut bacteria and leaky gut syndrome lead to more severe COVID-19. Good gut bacteria, it is speculated, are protective against viral infections, so it may be an excellent idea to repair and boost your gut bacteria if needed.

Since 2008, the Argentine government has provided 300,000 children with the probiotics Lactobacillus rhamnosus CRL 1505 isolated from goat's milk. This treatment has cut their respiratory infection rate by 50 percent. As a result, they also saw 61 percent fewer cases of tonsillitis and pharyngitis in the children.[44] Likewise, in Finland, CRL 1505 has been used extensively and safely with preterm babies and pregnant mothers. In people with leaky gut and those who are immune-compromised, there are warning labels attached to CRL

1505 use. More beneficial for them would be to use naturally fermented vegetables.

It may be difficult to understand why we need bacteria, often associated with adverse health, to maintain a healthy body. That's because good bacteria keep us healthy. On good bacteria, we are co-dependents and have symbiotic synergy. They are essential to us in the digestive process because they break down food, releasing nutrients to be bioavailable. The body's nutritional state is therefore reliant upon them for optimal function, as is the brain.

Unfortunately, good gut bacteria are constantly under attack from our food supply. Mass-produced foods such as dairy, beef, pork, and chicken are filled with residual antibiotics and other chemicals, as is our water supply with fluoride and chlorine.

Preserved food such as deli meats, sausages, bacon, and some forms of alcohol all have nitrates, which kill bacteria. Eating these foods assaults our gut bacteria, further complicated by taking antibiotics for minor reasons—certainly, another reason to eat a clean diet from humanly raised and organically certified food sources.

Regrettably, it is now out of fashion in the U.S. to eat fermented foods which contain high probiotics levels. My grandmother and probably your grandmother's table included many probiotic foods, such as fermented cabbage and other vegetables. Unfortunately, the only sauerkraut likely eaten today comes from a can and tops a Reuben sandwich.

The good news is, there are jars of sauerkraut or kimchee in the health food store's refrigerated department. Buy it and eat it. This will supply loads of lactobacillus and other beneficial bacteria. Make sure they are refrigerated and NOT made with vinegar, which inhibits bacterial growth. If you're making a face at the thought of this, so am I, but I find it tolerable to spread 1 or 2 tablespoons over food. I can hardly taste it. And surprisingly, sauerkraut juice, an elixir in health spas, is sort of delicious. It is also a good idea to bolster probiotics with foods that support good bacteria growth, such as raw green beans, raw asparagus, onion, leeks, garlic, and Jerusalem artichoke root if found. Both cooked asparagus, onion, and green beans are good, but the less cooked, the better. A tidbit: peel and eat the skin of an apple daily, another great prebiotic.

Every culture and ethnicity are shaped by geography and by the foods available in the region. Almost every one of them has created dishes that supply their need for good bacteria nutrition. Make it a point to include probiotics in your diet. They are the beginning of health

Iodine, as we discussed, is an essential part of a healthy diet. It drives the master gland, the thyroid. The average American gets about 150 mcg of iodine in their daily diet. The Japanese, on the other hand, ranking seventh as one of the healthiest countries, get 13,500 mcg daily. Three major bodies of water surround it, so their food supply includes eating seaweed and sea vegetables growing in saltwater and vegetables grown in iodine-rich soil. Besides, they eat a lot of sushi or other fish and shellfish that add to their natural iodine intake.

The geographic influences between the cuisines of Japan, Korea, Vietnam, China, and Thailand, remind me of the differences between Spanish, Italian, and French cooking, geographically connected countries. In each region, they are alike but different and unique. Kimchee, the pickled vegetables, cabbage, or green onion with red chilies eaten by the Koreans supply significant amounts of probiotics. The same is true of Japanese pickled vegetables made from daikon radish and turnips, providing a natural form of probiotics. A similar food in parts of Europe is sauerkraut. A serving of sauerkraut can have 100 times the amount of lactobacillus compared to a capsule. Fascinated with health, I decided to go around the world in my kitchen by creating dishes that offered meal variety and education stimulation. Travel with me to find your health.

CHAPTER TWENTY-ONE

EATING MY WAY AROUND
THE WORLD—HOW I STAY MOTIVATED WITH
CREATIVE COOKING

One of the reasons why most people revert to bad food is eating the same thing every day. A lack of variety and creativity in foods was my biggest enemy, so I spent time recreating foods from my travels or research. Food, good food, is the body's best defense. Since the beginning of my career, I've been more interested in how to eat to prevent disease than any other aspect of medicine. I have read hundreds of books on nutrition, and food and cooking is my hobby. I opt for eating the most nutritious foods, the superfoods, daily. When you eat right, your energy levels soar. The following advice on food is primary grain and sugar-free, yet you'll note I recommend a big diversity of foods to eat to stop you from falling off the wagon.

Living in the desert has brought new creativity to my cooking. I especially pay attention to fermented food and probiotic vegetables as they are the beginning of the body's nourishment. I make my cooking fun by going around the world in my kitchen! Join me.

From the Japanese, I have learned to undercook fish, particularly wild-caught Alaskan and Canadian salmon. They can also be eaten raw (sushi, sashimi). Since I'm 75 miles from the nearest sushi restaurant, I make it at home and use mung bean noodles in place of rice. I serve it with wasabi and ginger slices. I use wild-caught salmon to make Ceviche also. I tend to favor the Japanese approach to a meal, a combination of meat, shellfish and fish, eaten simultaneously. I love a Japanese breakfast of fish, mung bean noodles, the fermented vegetables daikon radish, an egg, miso soup, and a few orange slices. This, in my opinion, is the "breakfast of champions." Compare that to our grab-and-go danish or bagel.

From the Chinese, I sauté watercress, vegetables, and meats or fish and make a great stir-fry. I eat it with mung bean cellophane noodles.

From Brazil, I enjoy one or two selenium-rich Brazil nuts and eat them for my thyroid health.

From the Caribbean, I boil plantains or yucca, also known by its other name, cassava, and serve it with olive oil and salt instead of eating a potato. However, be aware, cassava is a thyroid-blocking food.

From Poland, I learned to make buckwheat grouts and mushrooms. From the Russians, borscht. From the Germans, I eat raw sauerkraut, which is worth repeating, has one hundred times as many lactobacilli as a probiotic capsule. From the Danish, I occasionally add blue cheese to a salad. From the Dutch, I thoroughly enjoy wintertime split pea soup with ham. From the French, I indulge in cooking with white wine and add mung bean sprouts to my salads, which were all the rage in Paris the last time I was there. On the occasion that a lobster finds its way to New Mexico, I make bisque from lobster shells thickened with potato starch, and yes, the dreaded cream is added. I'm glad we only find them occasionally. I make venison, buffalo, or elk in a burgundy wine sauce.

Salads are by far a favorite food. I am early to the farmers market to get fresh produce in the summer. I add shredded carrots, sprouts and other raw vegetables such as purple or green onions to most salads. I make a salad dressing, a ¼ cup of olive oil, hazelnut oil, and lemon. My top choice of seasoning is Vogel Herbamare, made in Switzerland with organic herbs and sea salt and a little kelp to add iodine. Mix that in with the salad dressing for the best possible salad. It's not just good, but great. Vogel Herbamare is sold in most health stores.

For me, the Italians inspire my everyday cooking and dinner parties. Eating risotto with porcini mushrooms is always a holiday treat. Most dishes are enhanced with tomatoes and Parmesan or Romano cheese; for example, a lentil soup becomes delicious when adding a tablespoon of Romano or the much more expensive Parmesan, but I am cautious with dairy products. I err on the side of lighter dishes such as asparagus cooked in olive oil with shredded Romano cheese and served with two eggs. Eggs, usually eaten at breakfast, make a great evening or supper food that's easily digested.

Mexican cooks have taught me that a squeeze of lime and a shot of hot sauce can make any soup, but especially a chicken soup, delicious. Fresh salsa and guacamole are always great and healthy. I add olive oil to the guacamole, and it becomes even more delicious because oil and fat enhance the taste of foods. I'm not suggesting eating salsa and guacamole with corn chips. Eating corn is something I avoid. Use plantain chips instead. Also, at Christmas here in New Mexico and elsewhere in the Hispanic world, they make Posole—from large corn kernels, known as hominy with pork and red chilies. If you've never had it, you are in for a treat. Find a Mexican restaurant during the holidays, and you should find it on the menu—fattening.

From the Irish, I dream about eating oatmeal, but since that's eating gluten, I have given it up, but I do miss it. I have learned to eat soup for breakfast from the Vietnamese and add raw vegetables such as thinly sliced green onion, cilantro, watercress, thinly sliced jalapeño and bean sprouts. From the Thai culture, I have learned the ancient art of making curry with coconut milk, vegetables and shrimp, but I don't eat it at night. Try it for lunch as spices can cause insomnia. The Spaniards give the celebration foods. Tortilla Española, a potato egg omelet, is made and served with Serrano ham on Christmas morning. The English have inspired me to cook a Christmas goose and save the goose fat to use later to sauté potatoes as the French do.

When I found myself in New York City on January 25, I searched for a restaurant serving a traditional Scottish Robert Burns' dinner and ate haggis. For the Arab world, I savor the elusive lamb's liver. Find it at an Arab butcher shop specializing in grass-fed lamb. From Lebanon, sesame paste known as Tahini is occasionally used in a salad dressing. From Israel, the wonderful ground sesame and honey-sweet Halvah, a Christmas time treat instead of all those cookies. From the Portuguese, I make bacalao—salted codfish.

I am a fan of great culinary dishes from Australia. Their fantastic, delicious ribs with a great barbeque sauce, is for me about the only reason to ever use sugar in cooking. As a matter of fact, put sugar on any meat, duck with orange sauce, Mongolian beef, Bulgogi adaptation from the Philippines, I'm hooked, and fall off the wagon and then have to fight my way off sugar yet again.

In the United States, regional foods are also appreciated. From New England, I enjoy shellfish and lobster. A real party around here is when we FedEx in lobsters and little neck clams. There are many squeals of happiness throughout the entire meal, not just for the party invitees but also for our bodies because we are feeding it iodine, selenium, and zinc. A hearty Cape Cod clam chowder thickened with potato starch is one of the most delicious soups ever. I am famous for this chowder. Buy a large frozen clam from Alaska. I always make it with a little dill as it's served at the Black Pearl in Newport, R.I.

Being from the Midwest, I still enjoy a summertime three-bean salad or sweet onion, cucumber, and tomato salad.

I'm beginning to like the new American cuisines from California with their exquisite salads, salad dressings. Classic and fantastic Caesar salad is a mainstay but use gluten-free croutons. California's gift to the world is found in most sushi restaurants, and is out of this world, California rolls sushi is served even in Japan and in my home on New Year's Eve.

From my mother's kitchen in Ohio, a summer dinner salad was occasionally made. She prepared a salad of wilted endive and escarole greens with bacon and eggs. The olive oil, vinegar and seasoning were heated and added to the greens, which she crunched with her hands, and topped with sliced hard-boiled eggs and bacon. Another wintertime dinner from her Slavic kitchen was to make stuffed cabbage and sauerkraut and kielbasa sausage, a meal that requires significant preparation. Today, however, that recipe has a shortcut. Just layer the different ingredients and cook.

From Jewish cuisine, I make chicken soup, the basis of winter cooking. Every two or three days, without much fuss into a pan, go spring water, chicken, garlic, onion, a few carrots, dried celery and parsley, a tomato from the freezer for flavor and potato to thicken it. The chicken itself goes to my dogs since I do not eat grain-fed anything, and it is cheaper to feed my dogs chicken than a decent can of dog food. Also, since I could have an obesity problem, if I let myself eat the standard American diet, my fat cells always seem to be waiting to turn themselves into rolls of fat. I fight the battle of the bulge daily; my biggest weapon is to cut the carbohydrates, and that cuts the cravings. My second biggest weapon is eating fatty meat for breakfast which cuts my carbohydrate craving for the rest of the day.

Spending each day trying to defeat the human body's desire to overeat all foods not good for us is exhausting. It's a small wonder that so many people fail and give in. The food battle becomes furious in the wintertime when we are designed to crave carbohydrates and pack on the pounds for the coming months of hibernation. I feel victorious when I diet my way thru December, and I don't gain the 5 to 10 lbs.

February and March are my battle months. It's as if my body says, "Now that the winter famine is almost over, you're not yet quite safe, so get out there and hunter-gather whatever food is available." This pattern is so distinct that

I watch for it, battle it, and still lose. I end up putting on the winter 5 lbs. because I cannot overcome the body's wisdom that this should be done for survival reasons. It is not unheard of to gain 10 lbs. during the holiday season, especially eating desserts. The benefits of being at your ideal weight are huge. We live healthier, longer, and happier lives if we cooperate with our bodies and give ourselves the proper nourishment.

When the menu calls for dessert, the Turks provide figs and dates crushed with walnuts or pecans to make a crushed pecan pie shell into which I pour a puree of raw berries, coconut milk, maple syrup or coconut crystals, and a layer of chocolate. When I am required to take food to a party, I opt for bringing this dessert. Sometimes I simply cut Halvah into sections. I buy them in the health store, ground sesame with brown rice syrup instead of sugar, and dip the top side into chocolate. They are a hit and always finished off. In the winter, for a dinner party dessert, I might make baked apple or pears in maple syrup, cinnamon, and walnuts; if decadence is required, it is easily found by adding a dollop of sour cream or heavy cream. A tablespoon of heavy cream will not do you in and will make the desert extra delicious. Finally, at Christmas, I make flan from Spain using honey.

FOOD AND HEALTH

Weekly I make a bison or grass-fed beef, or elk, super burger. First, I sauté an onion (shallots), garlic in olive oil, then add ground meat mixture of liver, heart and ribeye. I eat this with a salad, and it is the perfect grain-free meal, travels well in a container to work, and can be eaten several days in a row.

For the meltdown of crazy carbohydrate candy bar craving, I eat seeds and or nuts, with a bit of honey or maple syrup or coconut crystals and sometimes with cocoa powder, which cuts my sugar craving.

There are plenty of good books on diet. I recommend the "Good Health Diet" written by Paul Jaminet, Ph.D., and his wife, Shou-Ching Jaminet, Ph.D. Both authors are scientists. Both became sick. They chose a regime of eating healthy foods instead of taking medications and healed their bodies. Other specialists in health and nutrition have recommended Jaminet's diet as well, and to my great pleasure, I realized that I had been eating Jaminet's way all along. It certainly has worked for me. There is an ample food variety suggested in my around-the-world cuisine so, get creative. Healthy foods can be delicious, so go ahead have some fun with creating memorable and healthy dishes. It may sound time-consuming to prepare these kinds of food, but there are many shortcuts.

I make shopping as much fun as I make eating. It's like an outing with benefits. I mainly shop in the farmer's market, Asian or organic and health food stores. My shopping list is like an eclectic painting. Buying food in the health store is expensive, but the idea of putting fewer chemicals in my body should trump that, and it is by far healthier and less costly than eating in restaurants every day.

My Recommended Starter Shopping List
Condiments

- Olive oil extra virgin in dark glass
- Coconut oil extra virgin cold press
- Avocado oil

- Herbamare seasoning
- Coconut crystals instead of sugar
- Ground pecans or hazelnuts
- Ground coconut. Make sure it's unsweetened
- Potato starch
- Olives
- Tomato sauce in a glass jar
- Sesame paste, Tahini
- Bee pollen, local
- Sea salt
- Fish sauce
- Mayonnaise made with either olive oil or avocado oil, extra virgin coconut oil and extra virgin olive oil.

Dairy

- Grass-fed butter (pasture)
- Eggs organic from the farmer's market, fresh eggs with golden yokes from pasture free-range chickens. Make into omelets with fine herbs, shallots, tomatoes, bacon, and a little cheese are just plain old fantastic and eaten only occasionally, not regularly.
- Cheese: Parmesan and Romano
- Plant-based yogurts, coconut and cashew, are decent tasting (I prefer coconut yogurts).

Meats

- Grass-fed beef, pasture-raised without injecting hormones and antibiotics

- Bison
- Lamb
- Chicken, pasture-raised for broth

Seafood

- Alaskan or Pacific Salmon
- Sardines, double layer in olive oil, or brine
- Oysters, canned in olive oil
- Halibut
- Cod
- Shrimp and scallops, wild caught

Sweeteners

- Coconut manna and coconut sugar
- Honey local unrefined
- Maple syrup

Beverages

- Cocoa powder
- Green tea leaves
- Loose tea or tea bags
- Herbal tea "Nightly Night" formula

Carbohydrates Replacements

- Mung bean- cellophane noodles
- Sweet potato noodles Thailand
- Sweet potatoes

- Japanese sweet potatoes
- Regular potatoes but only a few and always organic
- Wild rice
- Plantains

Seasonings

- Dried red chilies, small ones
- Garlic
- Green onions
- Shallots for sautéing
- Yellow or white onions for soup
- Vidalia and purple onions for salads

NUTS

- Pumpkin seeds
- Sunflower seeds
- Walnuts
- Pecans
- Brazil nuts
- Almonds
- Hazelnuts
- Macadamia
- Cashew nuts

Vegetables

- Carrots
- Asparagus

- Swiss chard
- Avocados
- Organic lettuces

Fruits, if you must, choose apples. You can eat to wean off a heavy carbohydrate and sugar diet.

- Apples organic
- Blueberries
- Raspberries
- Cantaloupes
- Prunes
- Goji berries
- Incan golden berries
- Pomegranate

Other

- Dark chocolate
- Hemp hearts

Juices

Forget juices in general. Here in the desert, we get fresh pomegranate once a year. Anyone who does not drink pomegranate juice is missing out. I once saw an Iranian woman roll a pomegranate on the table with considerable pressure for a minute or two and then puncture it and squeezed the juice into a glass. I knew I was watching something which had been done for a millennium. I do the same thing and am rewarded with amazing nutrition. The fruit is loaded with vitamin C, aids digestion, is cancer-preventing, has antioxidants, anti-inflammatory properties, helps arthritis, heart disease, and so much more. In other words, it's a superfruit.

Kombucha: Try to find those made without sugar but rather sweetened slightly with fruit juice. At the risk of repeating myself too much, take note: probiotic-containing food must be refrigerated to keep the bacteria alive.

Ginger: Ginger is great for digestion. Make a lovely ginger tea from fresh ginger.

Lemon or limes or lemon juice or lime juice: Add it to your water, hot or cold. Lemon helps keep up hydration, is an excellent source of vitamin C, supports weight loss, improves skin quality, freshens the breath, aids in digestion, and helps prevent kidney stones. However, be careful as lemon juice is associated with dental erosion, so drink quickly and avoid sipping.

Note: There is no alcohol on the list. When I drink wine with food, I've noticed I eat more, so I don't do it, except when I'm hypnotized at a restaurant or dinner party, and then I regret it. I leave alcohol alone since it is just another way to gain weight, get dehydrated and interfere with a night of sleep. Drinking alcohol is also associated with breast cancer. The liver gets preoccupied with metabolizing alcohol which uses the same pathway for metabolizing estrogen. The alcohol wins, and estrogen levels are higher. The other cancers associated with alcohol consumption are the mouth, throat, voice box, esophagus, stomach, liver, colon, and rectum. In the medical community, there is beginning to be a reversal. Now it is said, and I believe it, that no amount of alcohol is healthy. Dealing with anxiety and using alcohol to treat the symptoms? Use cannabis.

CHAPTER TWENTY-TWO

MAKING IT BETTER FOR EVERYONE—
PERSONAL PROTECTION EQUIPMENT AND
THE VACCINE

Wearing protective gear is no child's play. Following the CDC's guideline on lessening contracting practices is a must. I repeat, it's a must. As part of a connected world, one does not have the right to ignore these CDC guidelines, and it is our duty as citizens to help minimize the spread of the deadly disease. Even as one mutation of virus wanes, another, more infectious variant is most likely on the way. It'll take some time to return to normal, and the new normal will require us to be prudent with the rules. Even if you think you're incapable of getting the virus or may survive it, you could become chronically ill, and of course, you are being socially irresponsible as you may pass it on to someone who might not survive or who will become chronically ill. You are responsible for your fellow man, and they are responsible for you.

- Wear masks that meet approved standards

- Wear gloves in situations where needed.
- Use alcohol-based sanitizers, lemons.
- Cover mouth when coughing
- Wash hands frequently and after touching public surfaces.
- Keep hands off the face.

Cover eyes with glasses or a face shield, especially health care workers.

Limit gatherings.

Not adhering to this general advice makes you potentially a deadly weapon. Using a face shield may be extreme for ordinary citizens, but why not err on the side of caution. We know the flu can enter through the eyes, and probably so can COVID-19. In Wuhan, China, they looked at hospitalized patients who wore glasses.[45] Out of 276 patients, only 5.8 percent were glass wearers compared to 32 percent of the population. JAMA, the Journal of American Association re Ophthalmology published this study and I quote, "SARS-CoV-2 was detected in tears or the conjunctival sacs of patients with COVID-19, and some ophthalmologists were reported to have been infected during routine treatment." Therefore, the eyes are considered a possible channel for SARS-CoV-2 to enter the human body.

Even as states open up, stay out of small rooms with other people, restaurants, cafes, airplanes and especially, breweries and bars, particularly if breakthrough infections increase. For those of us who want to make sure our favorite neighborhood restaurant remains viable, order take-out. If, however, your mental status depends on having dinner with a few friends, please follow PPE restaurant etiquette:

- Wear a mask when not eating.
- When entering and exiting, wear a mask!
- Wear a mask when walking to the restroom and while in the restroom.
- Keep the mask on while speaking to waitstaff; remember, they need protection just as much as you do.
- Wear the mask during the before and after dinner conversation. Or better yet, get restaurant food by takeout, as we know that restaurants are hot spots.
- Vaccine? Yes! Being vaccinated against COVID-19 is essential. For those with Long COVID, a vaccine can reactivate the immune system to do another round of cleaning up. So do yourself a favor and get vaccinated.

ANOTHER WORD ABOUT VACCINES

As of this writing, several vaccines are available to help stem the infection rates of COVID-19 and provide immunity. I'm not a big proponent of carte blanche vaccines which I believe the healthy body does not need, but it is certainly indicated in cases where the population is vulnerable. I am a proponent of the educated patient and want to share how vaccines help the immune system.

To best understand, let us first look at the healthy body's reaction to fighting viral or bacterial illnesses. When germs invade our bodies, they quickly attack our healthy cells and multiply rapidly. Immediately, our immune system goes into action flooding the infected area with white blood cells, the fighters of infection. Different types of white blood cells, of which there are three, respond differently to infections. Macrophages swallow up the germs, B-lymphocytes attack the virus, and T-lymphocytes attack the cells that have been affected by the virus. These activities leave behind antigens and antibodies, which are like a memory of the virus or bacteria, so we build resistance to a new virus invasion.

Currently, there are three vaccines for COVID-19. Each uses different methods, but all are intended to offer protection against the virus. In addition, vaccines work with the immune system to produce antibodies in people who did not get the virus, so they too can reduce the risk of getting a full-blown case of COVID-19 if later exposed. It appears that vaccines are also helping long-haulers. In their case, I vote yes, get vaccinated and see if you're one of the lucky ones who get better.

CHAPTER TWENTY-THREE

MAKING IT BETTER—FORTIFY YOUR THYROID HORMONE PRODUCTION AND STOP BLOCKING IT

These last two chapters of the book are dedicated to the all-powerful thyroid gland. One, because a thyroid malfunction (hypothyroidism) is a significant disease in America, and COVID-19's impact on it can be significant. Recently, and just before this book went to print, the CDC has recommended a thyroid workup for Long Covid Syndrome and two blood tests, TSH, Free T4. However, I am recommending a full panel TSH, Free T3, Free T4, rT3 and TPO antibodies. Again, a home blood spot test kit might give a more accurate picture of your thyroid status. If you recall, this master gland's hormones cut a wide swath in influencing most of the body's systemic functions: the heart, the muscles and digestive functions, brain development, gastrointestinal, reproductive system, bone maintenance etc. and the all-important immune system and regulates the body's metabolic rate. It is our energy system. It should be noted the immune system antibodies have a direct receptor for the thyroid hormone.

During the COVID-19 infection, the Italians figured out that the thyroid is also malfunctioning and, in some cases, directly attack the lungs, nose, brain, heart, kidneys, pancreas, gall bladder, and arteries.

Sadly, in general, thyroid-related diseases are often ignored in the American practice of medicine. Sixty percent of the people experiencing a thyroid problem are undiagnosed, which is astonishing.[46] Problems with the thyroid are usually caused by iodine deficiency, autoimmune diseases, genetic predispositions, among other conditions. Other significant causes are environmental insults to the body, such as mold and other pollutants.

Diagnosing thyroid insufficiency can be tricky. It usually starts with a TSH test that is typically normal; however, that result is erroneous. The challenge is understanding that a "normal" TSH thyroid test does not rule out a thyroid problem. Plus, the standard test for thyroid, the first one ordered, the TSH, isn't even a thyroid hormone but a pituitary hormone; go figure. This is one of the great paradoxes of our time. The two most prescribed medications before thyroid meds are for hypertension and cholesterol. However, elevated blood pressure and high cholesterol are the first warning signs that the thyroid gland is under stress. The leading cause of death, heart disease, according to a Harvard study, is associated with insufficient thyroid levels and elevated cholesterol levels, leading to hardening of the arteries, cardiovascular disease, atrial fibrillation and congestive heart failure.[47]

So dear patient, since the statistics for undiagnosed thyroid disease, 60 percent is so high, a lot is left up to you if you know something is not quite right with your health. Evaluate how you feel whether you have been diagnosed or not. Some of the most common hypothyroidism symptoms are fatigue, hair loss, dizziness, depression, brain fog, fibromyalgia, which means painful muscles and joints and a general feeling of unwellness. If it quacks like a duck, it is a duck. To rule out having a compromised Thyroid, ask the doctor to run a TSH, Free T3, Free T4 and rT3. If the test is positive, count the lucky stars because you're on your way to recovery with thyroid replacement hormone. However, if it is negative and your doctor repeats the most famous words in medicine, "It's not your thyroid," investigate it further by ordering a thyroid panel, home blood spot kit. They appear to give more accurate results. If symptoms persist, ask them to recheck the hormone levels. They are almost always borderline low. Low levels are an indication that boosting and working on thyroid health is indicated. As Dr. Jeffery Garber, M.D., a Harvard-affiliated endocrinologist, says, "More than half the people with normal thyroid function have symptoms of hypothyroidism."

Acting prophylactically means strengthening the thyroid's performance to produce the energy needed to help fight the virus, COVID-19. As you now know, the immune system requires a host of nutrients, minerals and trace elements, as discussed in the chapter on nutrients. If the pesky thyroid does not respond to an improved diet, supplements and vitamin D sunlight therapy, it may have to be supplemented for a while or permanently with replacement hormones. In COVID-19, because the thyroid can also be affected, it is good to be vigilant about checking your hormone levels. It's unlikely that a conventional provider will place a patient with a negative result on thyroid hormone replacement, even if the thyroid numbers are almost low as providers don't go against the holy grail of lab tests. So here again are the key elements to make sure you have in your diet as they are required for the body's synthesis. Vitamin D and vitamin B12, the cell factory, the mitochondria need magnesium. Other thyroid hormone requirements include zinc, selenium, iron, copper, folic acid—Vitamins A, B6, C, E, and, most importantly, iodine. Let's make sure the body has a good store of these vital vitamins, minerals, and thyroid hormones. Don't forget the sun, as a most positive ally. Everything recommended here strengthens the thyroid function. Know that frequent infections such as colds and flu, urinary tract infections, and in days past, Tuberculosis are common in people with hypothyroidism.

An additional thing I'd like to mention here about hormone deficiencies for conventional physicians: If your patient's best efforts to aid their recovery from COVID-19 fail, it may be time for them to consult with an Integrative Functional Medicine Doctor. It appears from the CDC list of labs reports that the problem for those with Long-Hauler Syndrome may be hormonal imbalance; in particular, low thyroid, low testosterone, and don't forget, low vitamin D, which is a hormone! Therefore, these missing hormones plus vitamin B12 must be corrected. Anti-aging Integrative Functional Medicine is a new specialty partially built around these very malfunctions of the hormonal system. If your personal care provider refers you to an endocrinologist, and you don't improve, seek out a Functional Integrative Medical provider.

We have spent a lot of time in *A Body Made to Win*, focusing on supporting the hormonal and immunological systems because they are that important to your health.

The 10 Commandments of Great Thyroid Health:

1. Exposure to sunlight activates thyroid hormone production. Thus, the sun is in control of our energy level. The increased energy level in the summer compared to the winter results from vitamin D exposure—active vs. hibernation is via thyroid hormone action.

2. Iodine: Since 3600 BC, the Chinese have used seaweed to cure thyroid disease, and similar recommendations are found in Hippocrates and Galen's writings. Kelp was the original source. By the 1920s in the US, iodine was added to salt to prevent hypothyroidism. Today, many people are using salt not fortified with iodine. It is essential to eat the right foods to help the body become more efficient at producing, storing, converting, and transporting thyroid hormones. Eat iodine-rich foods such as wild-caught seafood, seaweed, some grass-fed meat, and wild-caught game. Consider using sea salt with iodine. You can't make thyroid hormones without iodine because the thyroid hormone is composed of iodine.

3. Promote a healthy liver by eating a diet naturally high in selenium and zinc to facilitate thyroid hormone conversion; seafood, healthy red meat, organs meats, and grass-fed butter are good sources.

4. Eat omega 3 rich foods: seafood, red meat, grass-fed butter, and healthy oils made from coconut, olive, and avocado. The cell wall becomes more flexible and allows nutrients and hormones to enter.

5. Eat a paleo diet, recommended in the medical literature, as the best diet to strengthen thyroid production.

6. The use of medicinal cannabis THC/CBD has a positive effect on the TSH test and may explain why cannabis has such a positive effect. It is enhancing thyroid hormone.

7. The right supplements from natural sources, and I emphasize a healthful diet rather than pills, pills, and more pills. Nevertheless, supplementation is essential if needed.

8. Sufficient levels of antioxidants and vitamins in food are required, and importantly, vitamins C and A are needed for thyroid production.

9. Sleep well: medicinal cannabis indicia will help

10. Thyroid hormone replacement: not easy to attain since the lab tests often come back "Normal." Now is a perfect time to use your home blood spot kit. In some states, Paloma health will send you a kit and offer telemedicine visits with a doctor who can prescribe thyroid hormone replacement. WOW!

I want to emphasize how important it is to enhance cell wall permeability with omega 3 so that thyroid hormone can pass into the cell and work on a cellular level. Also, avoid the wrong foods, which block thyroid production and foods full of estrogen, which block thyroid transport to the cells. Also, avoid the foods that cause inflammation and allergy and stimulate the autoimmune attack on the thyroid gland, Hashimoto's, all previously discussed.

CHAPTER TWENTY-FOUR

THE ELEVEN OBSTACLES THYROID HORMONE HAS TO OVERCOME

Having a functioning thyroid is the key to good health. In the world we live today, there are many challenges the thyroid must overcome to remain healthy. These obstacles are ones most of us are not aware of and the reason why hypothyroidism is so pervasive. To promote thyroid health, watch out for these eleven impediments to optimal thyroid function.

There's an interesting statistic; the more hours you work, the more you increase your risk of developing hypothyroidism and herein lies the problem that gives rise to much of what we discuss below.

1. Stress calls into play a fight or flight response that is not sustainable...yet daily stress from the rat race life we lead today leaves us unhealthy. Chronic stress has a negative effect on our thyroid, T4 and T3 levels drop, and TSH rises, and weight gain follows. High levels of cortisol, elevated in stress, will eventually affect your thyroid function.

2. A bad diet is a recipe for thyroid disaster. Understanding thyroid function is an easier way to understand the important relationship between diet and food: The reason you feel so well when you've eaten a healthy diet is that you've given the energy system, i.e., the thyroid, everything it needs to make you energetic. (Go ahead, have some pancakes and fall asleep, and then tell me food doesn't affect energy.) And to boost energy further, what to do? I hope you know the answer: Be in the sun. Depleted energy is what comes from a bad diet. A deficiency of iodine, selenium and zinc causes a defect in the production and conversion of T4 storage hormone to T3 active hormone. With a chronic deficiency of these minerals, the thyroid gland cannot produce an adequate supply of thyroid hormones. The immune system tries its best to correct this deficiency by attacking the thyroid gland. It liberates T4, which goes into circulation to be converted to T3. Unfortunately, this is a disease process, Hashimoto's Thyroiditis, and little by little, year by year, thyroid production drops because antibodies from the immune system continue attacking the thyroid causing cellular death. Because the thyroid gland can also be undergoing a sudden super attack, you can lose energy all of a sudden, over a few weeks, as I think occurs with COVID Long Haulers.

What can you do to help? Make sure you have adequate minerals and elements required in your diet and feed your thyroid gland everything it needs. Remove foods that help provoke the attack; eggs, dairy, and particularly gluten, to name the top three. Lack of plant foods in the diet is also an issue. If vegetables, nuts, and seeds are not a regular food group in your diet, please correct this. A deficiency of plant food in the diet will result in a low magnesium state, which is the essential mineral to run the mitochondria, the cell factory that produces energy.

Natural Food Inhibitors: Avoid soy milk and soy products because they contain chemicals that prevent iodine from attaching (sorry, since tofu is wonderful stuff) to their receptors. Certain vegetables, such as broccoli, kale, and other cruciferous vegetables, will interfere with thyroid production and cause low thyroid function. Nutrient deficient food supply injected with pesticides, fertilizers, and other chemicals and hormones are major assaults on the thyroid. Also, stop eating foods that have estrogen in them. GMO foods are to be eaten under no circumstance. To do its work, the thyroid has to bind to the protein transport system to get to the cells. Being a pushy hormone, estrogen will knock the Thyroid Hormone off and instead bind itself to this transport protein. Therefore, prescription estrogen and estrogen found in dairy, chicken, and meats, bind to these transport proteins and block the receptor, thus lowering thyroid function. Dairy can contain 30 to 60 times the estrogen found in other foods due to milk produced from pregnant cows. It is capable of causing gynecomastia (men growing breast tissue).

3. Environmental Toxins: extended exposure to toxins can cause endocrine disruption. They are found in everyday things…Molds, waterproof clothing, non-stick cookware, fragrances, foods, beauty products, plastics and on and on…opt for all-natural products.

4. Lack of Sunlight. Sufficient vitamin D levels from sunlight exposure are required for thyroid production. It is not easy to overcome vitamin D deficiency. You'll have to work at it. A pill of synthetic vitamin D may seem to be a solution, but it is a very inferior solution compared to being in the sun.

5. Overuse of Supplements: Avoid supplements that block thyroid action, such as too much iodine, zinc, and selenium. These high-powered supplements can worsen hypothyroidism. Using foods rich in these minerals is the best source instead of taking supplements.

6. Replacement Thyroid Hormones: Let's imagine you can get thyroid hormone replacement. First, be aware that there are two types of replacement hormones: synthetic thyroid, levothyroxine and Cytomel, and dessicated animal porcine thyroid (almost bioidentical to human thyroid). Sometimes thyroid hormones can help the thyroid recover, and if it does, supplemental hormones can be discontinued. This usually occurs in the young. Older people will find themselves on the thyroid replacement for life. Naturally desiccated thyroid (NDT) is my choice and what I take and prescribe to my patients if indicated. It has been prescribed for 130 years and is a truly tried and true medication.

7. Conversions: There is a defect caused by hypothyroidism converting Beta-Carotene to vitamin A. This is important because vitamin A is needed to regulate thyroid production. Eating Vitamin, A rich vegetables with a good source of oil, such as olive oil, enhances the absorption of vitamin A. Sometimes

hypothyroid sufferers have yellowish skin, especially noted on the hands due to an accumulation of beta-carotenes that didn't get converted into vitamin A. Another conversion is T4 to T3, which occurs in the liver and stomach. It may be noted in alcohol drinkers, so don't wear out your liver with alcohol, which unfortunately is cytotoxic to the liver gland, which unfortunately means killing cells.

8. Cell Permeability: Cell receptors have to allow Thyroid Hormone, T3, to act on billions of little cell factories and mitochondria in every body system. Eating the American industrialized corn-fed animals (unhealthy themselves), coupled with a low-fat diet, having Essential Fatty Acid deficiency, create a shabby, inferior lipid membrane encompassing the cell. Thyroid Hormone then can't get in, and insulin can't pass either, which causes Type I and II diabetes. According to another great thyroid doctor, Mark Starr, M.D., this causes a similar condition with thyroid hormone, Type II Hypothyroidism. Both diseases are known to cause obesity.

9. Lack of sleep is associated with many bad things, probably because it is a symptom of low thyroid hormones.

10. Alcohol, toxic to the thyroid, kills its cells and is associated with lower circulating thyroid hormone levels.

11. Smoking tobacco is toxic to the thyroid and is associated with hypothyroidism

A bonus: Get your thyroid tested as part of your routine health maintenance.

If you are experiencing thyroid symptoms, I suggest three books that are written with the patient in mind.

The three books which have had the greatest impact on me and may offer you some insights are Broda Barnes, M.D., *Hypothyroidism the Unsuspected Illness*. Mark Starr, M.D, *Hypothyroidism Type Two*, and Stephen Langer, M.D, *Solved: The Riddle of Illness*.

I thank these doctors for their fine work, as considering its enormous impact on health in so many medical curricula, the importance of this little butterfly organ is not stressed.

A bonus: Get your thyroid tested as part of your routine health maintenance.

CONCLUSION

This book used COVID-19 to discuss the body's ability to win against disease and heal itself from an attack by a pathogen and other diseases, no matter the cause or origin of the malady. I hope through this book you've come to appreciate the most incredible and intelligent creation ever designed —a body made to win. The human body built to heal itself—a creation in which the most minute detail was considered, is your best asset. It clearly suggests that Mother Nature is the boss and makes no mistakes.

The body's interconnectivity, interdependence and symbiotic relationship with the environment is something to marvel about. Yet, so many of us take it for granted. As holistic medical practitioners, we fully appreciate that balancing individuals' overall physical, mental, emotional, and spiritual well-being is necessary before deciding on a course of or recommending treatments.

Now that you're at the end of the book, like me, I hope you agree and have come to appreciate that good medicine must treat the body as a complex, integrated system. If we treat the body with the respect it deserves, it will lead us on a path of optimizing our health to a long, happy and fruitful life.

The trend in medicine toward super subspecialties needs to better appreciate that every part of the body is dependent on every other part. If one part isn't working, most likely, it's affecting something else, and the entire body goes out of balance. My approach to holistic healing is nothing new. Natural medicine has been practiced for centuries.

At the Hot Springs Wellness Center, indeed, we consider the entire being—body, mind, and spirit, in our quest to find the best solutions to health and wellness. The overall health of a person is their greatest asset.

As I mentioned throughout this book, as a doctor, I will assess health options and recommend the best opportunities for healing from conventional medication to alternative therapies for my patients. Still, in my almost thirty-eight years of practicing medicine, I have found that many diseases can be treated without invasive treatments. However, thyroid hormone replacement, in many cases, will be required.

I hope you have been motivated to take control of your health and find interest in being an informed patient ready to fully participate in your own healing. Below I have outlined the principles we follow at the Hot Springs Wellness Center. They are the Principles of Holistic Medicine, much like the Hippocratic oath I took as a medical doctor upon graduation from medical school.

Principles of Holistic Medicine

Holistic medicine believes that individuals are ultimately responsible for their own health and well-being. Often a loving and supporting environment holds the space for patients looking to radically and permanently take charge of their health and well-being.

Other principles of holistic medicine include the following:

- All people have innate healing powers.
- A patient is a person, not a disease.
- Healing takes a team approach involving the patient and doctor and addresses aspects of a person's life using *all* available healthcare options.
- Treatment involves fixing the cause of the condition, not just alleviating the symptoms.
- Recovery often requires a significant effort on the patient's part.

ACKNOWLEDGEMENTS

Thank you to all the amazing people who rallied around during the writing and publication of this book. I would like to thank the following people for their support while writing this book: Gordon Edelheit, Robin Love, Nicolette Love, Ph.D., Louise Masingale, assistant, Dorcas Brem, LPCC, Catherine Wright, Associate Professor Writing and Rhetoric, Middlebury College, Jasna Brown, Caroline George, Ramon Saavedra, M.D., Julia R. Rackow, media specialist, Davey Packard, IT, Mo Hollis and Nikki Caputo, videographers, Bob Lamb, and my publisher the fabulous, stupendous, you can't stop this woman so don't try, Marva Allen. To my editor Winsome Hudson, thanks for enhancing the work with points of language and clarity. For the people who generously provided a blurb for the book, Dr. Kenneth Silvestri, Ricardo Rubio, M.D., Jim English, Founder and Owner, Tango Advanced Nutrition, thank you. Special thanks to Dr. Paulette Moulton for writing the Foreword.

GLOSSARY

ADD: Attention Deficit Disorder

ADHD: Attention Deficit Hyperactivity Disorder (adults)

AIDS: Acquired Immunodeficiency Syndrome

ALZHEIMERS: A progressive disease that destroys memory and other important mental functions.

CBD: Cannabidiol, commonly known as Cannabis

CDC: Center for Disease Control and Prevention

COPD: Chronic Obstructive Pulmonary Disease

COVID-19: is a contagious disease caused by severe acute respiratory syndrome coronavirus 2 (SARS-CoV-2).

ESS: Empty Sella Syndrome is a disorder of the bony structure surrounding the pituitary gland.

FDA: Food and Drug Administration

H1N1: A subtype of the Influenza A virus commonly known as the Swine Flu

LONG HAULERS: Colloquial: People with lingering illness after COVID-19. Brain fog, compromised breathing, headaches, insomnia, fatigue persists even after recovery.

NEJM: New England Journal of Medicine

NIH: National Institute of Health

OTC: Over the Counter Drugs

TAMIFLU: An anti-viral drug for the Flu virus

THC: The Psychoactive Compound in Cannabis

TCM: Traditional Chinese Medicine

WHO: World Health Organization

Z-PAK: Zithromax is a powerful antibiotic for bacterial infections.

INDEX

Understanding How COVID-19 Vaccines Work | CDC
https://www.cdc.gov › vaccines › how-they-work   *page* 9

11. Analgesics in the Treatments for COVID-19 – Harvard
Health Publishing https://www.health.harvard.edu ›
diseases-and-conditions.   *page* 13

12. Fever | Main Line Health | Philadelphia, Pennsylvania
https://www.mainlinehealth.org › conditions › fever. Is
temperature a good marker for COVID-19? https://
www.capecodhealth.org › coronavirus › is-tempera...
https://www.health.harvard.edu   › diseases-and-
conditions   *page* 14

13. Physicians at the Royal Society of Medicine in London
do not recommend that patients lower their fever at the
beginning of a COVID-19 infection   *page* 14

14. Fever – Symptoms and causes – Mayo Clinic https://
www.mayoclinic.org   *page* 14

15. When monitoring for COVID-19 symptoms, what
temperature is considered a fever? https://www.
capecodhealth.org   *page* 15

16. Mapped:The6,000-YearHistoryofMedicalCannabis.https://
www.visualcapitalist.com;   https://www.forbes.com/sites/
emilyearlenbaugh/2020/07/21/new-research-suggests-ter-
penes-and-cbd-work-3xs-better-for-covid-19-inflamma-
tion-than-corticosteroid/?sh=68f5e8534e95   *page* 22

17. COVID-19: Potential Causes for Hypoxemia | Loyola
Medicine. https://loyolamedicine.org   *page* 25

18. Mortality Analyses - Johns Hopkins Coronavirus Resource. https://coronavirus.jhu.edu *page* 27

19. COVID-19 and Flu testing in fall https://www.cdc.gov/coronavirus/2019-ncov/lab/multiplex.html *page* 27

20. Human Metapneumovirus Clinical Features | CDC. https://www.cdc.gov *page* 27

21. Spike in People Dying at Home. https://www.propublica.org *page* 28

22. Pulmonary Fungus Infections Associated with Steroid and https://journal.chestnet.org › article › fulltext *page* 30

23. Vitamin D Deficiency in COVID-19 Quadrupled Death Rate. https://www.medscape.com: https://www.medscape.com/viewarticle/942497 Relationship between fever and pulse rate https://academic.oup.com/qjmed/article-abstract/os-20/78/205/1515205?redirectedFrom=PDF *page* 30

24. Sunlight increases testosterone/Sunbathing can boost men's sex drive https://www.hindustantimes.com *page* 37

25. Territorial Medicine - Albuquerque Historical Society. https://albuqhistsoc.org https://www.cdc.gov/global-health/newsroom/topics/tb/index.html *page* 39

26. Vitamin D Deficiency and Tuberculosis Progression: https://www.ncbi.nlm.nih.gov › articles › PMC2954005: *page* 40

27. The Protective Role of Astaxanthin for UV-Induced Skin https://www.ncbi.nlm.nih.gov *page* 40

28. Turkey: Renaissance of Thermal Therapy https://www. magazine.medicaltourism.com   *page* 41

29. https://globalriskinsights.com/2017/04/radar-traditional-chinese-medicine-became-one-africas-fastest-growing   *page* 53

30. Who estimates https://africacheck.org/fact-checks/reports/do-80-s-africans-regularly-consult-traditional-healers-claim-unproven   *page* 53

31. TCM in Italy: https://www.thestar.com.my/opinion/columnists/colours-of-china/2020/03/30/tcms-role-in-covid-19-treatment   *page* 54

32. Potential COVID-19 drug azithromycin may increase risk for dimentuahttps://www.sciencedaily.com   *page* 58

33. WHO recommends against the use of remdesivir in COVID-19. https://www.who.int   *page* 59

34. Remdesivir for the Treatment of COVID-19. NEJM for COVID-19. https://www.healthline.com   *page* 59

35. Oral medication in pill from Pfizer. https://www.very-wellhealth.com/pfizer-developing-covid-19-at-home-treatment-pill-5184029. https://pubmed.ncbi.nlm.nih.gov/32380291/   *page* 60

36. Doctors warn that sugar can temporarily weaken your immune. www.cnet.com   *page* 61

37. https://www.cnbc.com/2020/04/15/drinking-alco-hol-can-make-the-coronavirus-worse-the-who-says-in-recommending-restricting-access.html   *page* 65

38. Alcohol Use and Cancer - American Cancer Society: https://www.cancer.org   *page* 65

39. Alcohol and COVID-19: what you need to know - WHO/Europe; https://www.euro.who.int   *page* 65

40. Debunking the health benefits of apple cider vinegar ... https://www.uchicagomedicine.org   *page* 70

41. Nutrition and Immunity. Examples of nutrients that have been identified as critical for the growth and function of immune cells include vitamin C, vitamin D, zinc, selenium, iron, and protein (including the amino acid glutamine). https://www.hsph.harvard.edu   *page* 71

42. Vegans, Vegetarians and Pescatarians Are at Risk of Iodine Deficiency in Norway. https://pubmed.ncbi.nlm.nih.gov/33233534/   https://www.ncbi.nlm.nih.gov/pmc/articles/PMC7699510   *page* 73

43. A Call for a Low-Carb Diet That Embraces Fat - The New York Times.https://www.google.com/amp/s/www.nytimes.com/2014/09/02/health/low-carb-vs-low-fat-diet.amp.html   *page* 75

44. Towards a better understanding of Lactobacillus rhamnosus. https://www.ncbi.nlm.nih.gov   *page* 75

45. Association of Daily Wear of Eyeglasses with Susceptibility. https://jamanetwork.com   *page* 95

46. https://www.hcplive.com/view/covid19-induced-thyroid-infection-identified-in-italian-patient   *page* 98

47. Up to 60 percent of those with thyroid disease are unaware of their condition. General Information/Press Room |

American Thyroid Association. https://www.thyroid.org › Media Hypothyroidism: The cardiac connection how-does-cardiovascular-disease-increase-the-risk-of-severe-illness-and-death-from-COVID-19-https://www.health.harvard.edu/heart-health/thyroid-hormone-how-it-affects-your-heart   *page* 98

Made in the USA
Las Vegas, NV
15 January 2023

65655398R00089